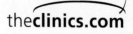

theclinics.com

SLEEP MEDICINE CLINICS

Sleep and Cardiovascular Disease

Guest Editor
SHAHROKH JAVAHERI, MD

December 2007 • Volume 2 • Number 4

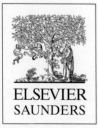

ELSEVIER
SAUNDERS

An imprint of Elsevier, Inc
PHILADELPHIA LONDON TORONTO MONTREAL SYDNEY TOKYO

W.B. SAUNDERS COMPANY
A Division of Elsevier Inc.

1600 John F. Kennedy Boulevard • Suite 1800 • Philadelphia, PA 19103-2899

http://www.sleep.theclinics.com

SLEEP MEDICINE CLINICS Volume 2, Number 4
December 2007 ISSN 1556-407X, ISBN-13: 978-1-4160-5123-7 ISBN-10: 1-4160-5123-6

Editor: Sarah E. Barth

The ideas and opinions expressed in *Sleep Medicine Clinics* do not necessarily reflect those of the Publisher. The Publisher does not assume any responsibility for any injury and/or damage to persons or property arising out of or related to any use of the material contained in this periodical. The reader is advised to check the appropriate medical literature and the product information currently provided by the manufacturer of each drug to be administered to verify the dosage, the method and duration of administration, or contraindications. It is the responsibility of the treating physician or other health care professional, relying on independent experience and knowledge of the patient, to determine drug dosages and the best treatment for the patient. Mention of any product in this issue should not be construed as endorsement by the contributors, editors, or the Publisher of the product or manufacturers' claims.

Sleep Medicine Clinics (ISSN 1556-407X) is published quarterly by W.B. Saunders Company, 360 Park Avenue South, New York, NY 10010-1710. Months of publication are March, June, September and December. Business and editorial offices: 1600 John F. Kennedy Boulevard, Suite 1800, Philadelphia, PA 19103-2899. Accounting and circulation offices: 6277 Sea Harbor Drive, Orlando, FL 32887-4800. Periodicals postage paid at New York, and additional mailing offices. Subscription prices are $139.00 per year (US individuals), $70.00 (US students), $303.00 (US institutions), $149.00 (Canadian individuals), $85.00 (Canadian students), $279.00 (Canadian institutions), $161.00 (foreign individuals), $92.00 (foreign students), and $326.00 (foreign institutions). Foreign air speed delivery is included in all *Clinics* subscription prices. All prices are subject to change without notice. POSTMASTER: Send address changes to *Sleep Medicine Clinics*, Elsevier Periodicals Customer Service, 6277 Sea Harbor Drive, FL 32887-4800. **Customer Service: 1-800-654-2452 (US). From outside of the United States, call 1-407-345-4000. E-mail: hhspcs@wbsaunders.com**.

Reprints: For copies of 100 or more, of articles in this publication, please contact the Commercial Reprints Department, Elsevier Inc., 360 Park Avenue South, New York, New York 10010-1710. Tel.: (212) 633-3813, Fax: (212) 462-1935, e-mail: reprints@elsevier.com.

Printed in the United States of America.

GOAL STATEMENT

The goal of *Sleep Clinics of North America* is to keep practicing physicians up to date with current clinical practice by providing timely articles reviewing the state of the art in patient care.

ACCREDITATION

The *Sleep Clinics of North America* is planned and implemented in accordance with the Essential Areas and Policies of the Accreditation Council for Continuing Medical Education (ACCME) through the joint sponsorship of the University of Virginia School of Medicine and Elsevier. The University of Virginia School of Medicine is accredited by the ACCME to provide continuing medical education for physicians.

The University of Virginia School of Medicine designates this educational activity for a maximum of 15 *AMA PRA Category 1 Credits*™. Physicians should only claim credit commensurate with the extent of their participation in the activity.

The American Medical Association has determined that physicians not licensed in the US who participate in this CME activity are eligible for 15 *AMA PRA Category 1 Credits*™.

Credit can be earned by reading the text material, taking the CME examination online at http://www.theclinics.com/home/cme, and completing the evaluation. After taking the test, you will be required to review any and all incorrect answers. Following completion of the test and evaluation, your credit will be awarded and you may print your certificate.

FACULTY DISCLOSURE/CONFLICT OF INTEREST

The University of Virginia School of Medicine, as an ACCME accredited provider, endorses and strives to comply with the Accreditation Council for Continuing Medical Education (ACCME) Standards of Commercial Support, Commonwealth of Virginia statutes, University of Virginia policies and procedures, and associated federal and private regulations and guidelines on the need for disclosure and monitoring of proprietary and financial interests that may affect the scientific integrity and balance of content delivered in continuing medical education activities under our auspices.

The University of Virginia School of Medicine requires that all CME activities accredited through this institution be developed independently and be scientifically rigorous, balanced and objective in the presentation/discussion of its content, theories and practices.

All authors/editors participating in an accredited CME activity are expected to disclose to the readers relevant financial relationships with commercial entities occurring within the past 12 months (such as grants or research support, employee, consultant, stock holder, member of speakers bureau, etc.). The University of Virginia School of Medicine will employ appropriate mechanisms to resolve potential conflicts of interest to maintain the standards of fair and balanced education to the reader. Questions about specific strategies can be directed to the Office of Continuing Medical Education, University of Virginia School of Medicine, Charlottesville, Virginia.

The authors/editors listed below have identified no professional or financial affiliations for themselves or their spouse/partner:
Miguel J. Arias, MD, PhD; W. de Backer, MD; Jean-Philippe Baguet, MD, PhD; Sarah Barth (Acquisitions Editor); Santiago Carrizo, MD; Jerome Dempsey, PhD; Karl A. Franklin, MD, PhD; Francisco Garcia-Rio, MD, PhD; Suraj Kapa, MD; Fotis Kapsimalis, MD; Meir Kryger, MD, FRCCP; Teofilo Lee-Chiong, Jr., MD (Consulting Editor); Patrick Levy, MD, PhD; Jose M. Marin, MD; Walter T. McNicholas, MD, FRCPI, FRCPC; Vahid Mohsenin, MD; Yannik Neuder, MD; Yüksel Peker, MD, PhD; Jean-Louis Pepin, MD, PhD; Renaud Tamisier, MD, PhD; and, Henry Yaggi, MD, MPH.

The authors/editors listed below identified the following professional or financial affiliations for themselves or their spouse/partner:
Donna L. Arand, PhD is an independent contractor for Cephalon, on the Speaker's Bureau for Sanofi and Takada and is a consultant for Jazz.
Heinrich F. Becker, MD serves on the Speaker's Bureau for Respironics, Heimen and Lowenstein, Weimmann and ResMed and serves on an Advisory Committee for ResMed.
Michael Bonnet, PhD is an independent contractor for Cephalon, is on the Speaker's Bureau for Sanofi and Takada and is a consultant for Jazz.
Jan Hedner, MD, PhD owns stock and is a patent holder for Cereum Science AB.
Shahrokh Javaheri, MD (Guest Editor) is an independent contractor, consultant, and on the Speaker's Bureau for Respironics, is on the Speaker's Bureau for Cephalon/Takeda/Res Med, is an independent contractor for Sanofi Aventis, is on the Speaker's Bureau for Sepacor/Boreige/Ingelheim and is a consultant for Nexan.
Virend K. Somers, MD, PhD is a consultant for Cardiac Concepts and has received research honorarium grant from Res Med and Res Med Foundation.

Disclosure of Discussion of non-FDA approved uses for pharmaceutical products and/or medical devices:
The University of Virginia School of Medicine, as an ACCME provider, requires that all faculty presenters identify and disclose any "off label" uses for pharmaceutical and medical device products. The University of Virginia School of Medicine recommends that each physician fully review all the available data on new products or procedures prior to instituting them with patients.

TO ENROLL

To enroll in the *Sleep Clinics of North America* Continuing Medical Education program, call customer service at 1-800-654-2452 or visit us online at www.theclinics.com/home/cme. The CME program is available to subscribers for an additional fee of $99.95.

SLEEP AND CARDIOVASCULAR DISEASE

CONSULTING EDITOR

TEOFILO LEE-CHIONG, Jr., MD
Head, Section of Sleep Medicine, National Jewish
Medical and Research Center, Denver; Associate
Professor of Medicine, University of Colorado
Health Sciences Center, Denver, Colorado

GUEST EDITOR

SHAHROKH JAVAHERI, MD
Professor Emeritus of Medicine, University
of Cincinnati College of Medicine, Cincinnati;
Medical Director, Sleepcare Diagnostics, Mason,
Ohio

CONTRIBUTORS

DONNA L. ARAND, PhD
Associate Research Professor of Neurology,
Wright State University School of Medicine,
Dayton; Wallace Kettering Neuroscience
Institute, Kettering, Ohio

MIGUEL A. ARIAS, MD, PhD
Cardiology Department, Hospital Virgen de la
Salud, Toledo, Spain

W. De BACKER, MD
Department of Pulmonary Medicine, University
Hospital Antwerp, Edegem, Belgium

JEAN-PHILIPPE BAGUET, MD, PhD
Professor in Cardiology, Cardiology and
Hypertension Clinics, Centre Hospitalier
Universitaire de Grenoble, Grenoble,
France

HEINRICH F. BECKER, MD
Professor of Medicine, Philipps-University
Marburg; Director, Division of Pulmonary and
Critical Care Medicine, AK Barmbek, Hamburg,
Germany

MICHAEL H. BONNET, PhD
Professor of Neurology, Wright State University
School of Medicine, Dayton; Wallace Kettering
Neuroscience Institute, Kettering, Ohio

SANTIAGO J. CARRIZO, MD
Respiratory Service, Hospital Universitario Miguel
Servet; University of Zaragoza, Zaragoza, Spain

J.A. DEMPSEY, PhD
Professor of Population Health Sciences, John
Rankin Laboratory of Pulmonary Medicine,
University of Wisconsin, Madison, Wisconsin

KARL A. FRANKLIN, MD, PhD
Associate Professor, Department of Pulmonary
Medicine, Norrland University Hospital, Umeå,
Sweden

FRANCISCO GARCÍA-RÍO, MD, PhD
Service of Pulmonary Medicine, Hospital
Universitario La Paz; Associate Professor of
Medicine, School of Medicine, Universidad
Autónoma de Madrid, Madrid, Spain

JAN HEDNER, MD, PhD
Professor of Sleep Medicine, Sleep Laboratory
Services, Department of Pulmonary Medicine,
Sahlgrenska University Hospital, Gothenburg,
Sweden

SHAHROKH JAVAHERI, MD
Professor Emeritus of Medicine, University of
Cincinnati College of Medicine, Cincinnati;
Medical Director, Sleepcare Diagnostics,
Mason, Ohio

SURAJ KAPA, MD
Division of Internal Medicine, Mayo Clinic
College of Medicine, Rochester, Minnesota

FOTIS KAPSIMALIS, MD
Associate Director, Department of Thoracic
Medicine, Sleep Laboratory, Henry Dunant
Hospital, Athens, Greece

MEIR KRYGER, MD, FRCCP
Director of Sleep Research and Education,
Gaylord Hospital, Wallingford; Clinical
Professor of Medicine, University of
Connecticut, Connecticut

PATRICK LÉVY, MD, PhD
Professor in Physiology, Inserm ERI 17, Hypoxia
Pathophysiology (HP2) Laboratory, Joseph
Fourier University; Sleep Laboratory, EFCR, Pôle
Rééducation et Physiologie, Centre Hospitalier
Universitaire de Grenoble, Grenoble, France

JOSE M. MARIN, MD
Respiratory Service, Hospital Universitario Miguel
Servet; and University of Zaragoza, Zaragoza,
Spain

WALTER T. McNICHOLAS, MD, FRCPI, FRCPC
Professor, Respiratory Sleep Disorders Unit, St.
Vincent's University Hospital; The Conway
Institute of Biomolecular and Biomedical
Research, University College Dublin, Ireland

VAHID MOHSENIN, MD
Professor, Section of Pulmonary and Critical
Medicine; Director, Yale Center for Sleep Medicine,
Yale University School of Medicine, New Haven,
Connecticut

YANNICK NEUDER, MD
Physician, Cardiology and Hypertension Clinics,
Centre Hospitalier Universitaire de Grenoble,
Grenoble, France

YÜKSEL PEKER, MD, PhD
Consultant Internist and Pulmonologist,
Department of Pulmonary Medicine,
Sahlgrenska University Hospital,
Gothenburg, Sweden

JEAN-LOUIS PÉPIN, MD, PhD
Professor in Physiology, Inserm ERI 17,
Hypoxia Pathophysiology (HP2) Laboratory,
Joseph Fourier University; Sleep Laboratory,
EFCR, Pôle Rééducation et Physiologie, Centre
Hospitalier Universitaire de Grenoble,
Grenoble, France

VIREND K. SOMERS, MD, PhD
Professor of Medicine, Division of Cardiovascular
Diseases and Internal Medicine, Mayo Clinic
College of Medicine, Rochester, Minnesota

RENAUD TAMISIER, MD, PhD
Assistant Professor in Physiology, Inserm ERI 17,
Hypoxia Pathophysiology (HP2) Laboratory,
Joseph Fourier University; Sleep Laboratory, EFCR,
Pôle Rééducation et Physiologie, Centre
Hospitalier Universitaire de Grenoble, Grenoble,
France

HENRY YAGGI, MD, MPH
Assistant Professor, Section of Pulmonary and
Critical Care Medicine, Clinical Epidemiology
Research Center, VA Connecticut Healthcare
System, West Haven; Section of Pulmonary and
Critical Medicine, Yale University School of
Medicine, New Haven, Connecticut

SLEEP AND CARDIOVASCULAR DISEASE

Volume 2 • Number 4 • December 2007

Contents

Poor sleep can have many connotations, and an examination of cardiovascular relationships must be done with reference to the various definitions of poor sleep. The most common connotation of poor sleep is insomnia. Sleep may be less than optimal for a number of additional reasons, however, including lack of opportunity, fragmentation, or stress not producing traditional insomnia. This article discusses each of these types of poor sleep. This article does not discuss the relationship of medical disorders that produce insomnia to cardiovascular disease.

The mechanisms underlying cardiovascular disease in patients with obstructive sleep apnea are still poorly understood. The pathogenesis is likely to be a multifactorial process involving a diverse range of mechanisms, including sympathetic nervous system overactivity, selective activation of inflammatory pathways, endothelial dysfunction, and metabolic dysregulation, the latter particularly involving insulin resistance and disordered lipid metabolism. This sleep breathing disorder is thought to contribute to, or be a cause of systemic hypertension, atherosclerosis, coronary artery disease, heart failure, atrial fibrillation, and stroke.

Obstructive sleep apnea (OSA) is an independent risk factor for systemic and pulmonary arterial hypertension. Sympathetic activation, caused by recurrent hypoxemia, is the most important pathomechanism for systemic hypertension, which is probably the most important link concerning the markedly increased mortality and morbidity in untreated OSA patients. Effective continuous positive airway pressure (CPAP) treatment substantially reduces blood pressure in hypertensive OSA patients. Similarly, recurrent hypoxemia causing pulmonary arteriolar vasoconstriction mediates development of pulmonary hypertension. Limited data suggest that use of CPAP improves pulmonary arterial hypertension.

Obstructive apneas during sleep lead to a sequence of events that independently, or in concert with other recognized risk factors, appear to induce harmful effects on vascular structure and function. Although the epidemiologic support for a causal relationship between obstructive sleep apnea (OSA) and coronary artery disease (CAD) is rapidly increasing, data is still not fully conclusive. In general, the relationship is stronger in clinical cohorts, compared with in the general population, suggesting that comorbid OSA may provide an additive or synergistic risk factor for development of CAD in obese, hypertensive, smoking, or hyperlipidemic subjects. Recognition of the adverse impact of OSA on vascular disease may open a perspective of new primary and secondary prevention models for CAD, involving identification and elimination of the sleep and breathing disorder.

There are some epidemiologic data that potentially implicate obstructive sleep apnea syndrome as a cause of left ventricular systolic and diastolic dysfunction. The main pathophysiologic mechanisms involved are the sympathetic overactivity, the alterations in left ventricular preload and afterload, and the effects of hypoxemia. This article considers the clinical implications of this relationship and reviews the available data on the efficacy of continuous positive airway pressure in patients with obstructive sleep apnea syndrome and left ventricular dysfunction.

There is a relationship between arrhythmias and sleep apnea, most notably during sleep. A common rhythm disturbance is nocturnal bradyarrhythmias that occur in association with apneic episodes; however, because of long-term autonomic, functional, and structural cardiac changes, in addition to decreased ischemic threshold, patients with sleep apnea may potentially be at higher risk for developing atrial fibrillation and ventricular arrhythmias. These complications of untreated sleep apnea may conceivably be implicated in nocturnal sudden cardiac death.

This article explores the relationship between obstructive sleep apnea syndrome and stroke by critically reviewing the current literature. First, epidemiologic studies are analyzed with respect to issues regarding the strength of the association, and the consistency of the association using different study designs and different populations. Next, the biologic plausibility of the relationship is explored by reviewing studies that examine the pathophysiology of sleep apnea and stroke. Subsequently, studies exploring the therapeutic impact of obstructive sleep apnea syndrome on stroke and cardiovascular risk are reviewed. Finally, public health implications are discussed.

Mortality in Obstructive Sleep Apnea

593

Jose M. Marin and Santiago J. Carrizo

Many recent prospective, long-term, controlled studies suggest that in untreated patients with sleep apnea, the risk of death from all-causes and particularly cardiovascular causes is increased. There is a relation between the severity of this disease and cardiovascular risk, but the effective treatment with nasal continuous positive airway pressure significantly reduces the mortality associated with this medical condition. This article examines the growing evidence that links obstructive sleep apnea with cardiovascular outcomes and specifically with an excess of mortality.

Obstructive Sleep Apnea in Pregnancy

603

Fotis Kapsimalis and Meir Kryger

During pregnancy several physical and hormonal alterations may affect normal sleep and the respiratory system and predispose pregnant women to the development of sleep-disordered breathing (SDB) or worsen pre-existing obstructive sleep apnea syndrome (OSAS). SDB has been associated with several complications of pregnancy affecting maternal and fetal health. Clinicians should evaluate more closely obese pregnant women and those who develop hypertension. Early recognition and treatment of SDB may improve the outcome of pregnancy but the indications for treatment of OSAS need to be investigated. The diagnosis of OSAS in pregnancy requires a high index of suspicion and prevention of suspected SDB should be incorporated in the management of pregnancy.

Prevalence and Impact of Central Sleep Apnea in Heart Failure

615

PatrickLévy, Jean-Louis Pépin, Renaud Tamisier, Yannick Neuder, Jean-Philippe Baguet, and Shahrokh Javaheri

Sleep apnea is commonly found in patients with systolic heart failure, and recent studies strongly suggest that the prevalence of central sleep apnea remains high, in spite of the use of contemporary treatment of heart failure, including beta-blockers. Furthermore, it has been shown that central sleep apnea may contribute to mortality of heart failure patients. However, the impact of therapy for sleep apnea on survival of heart failure patients needs to be further determined.

Mechanisms of Sleep Apnea and Periodic Breathing in Systolic Heart Failure

623

Shahrokh Javaheri and J.A. Dempsey

Periodic breathing and central sleep apnea are common in patients with systolic heart failure. The mechanisms of central sleep apnea are complex. Recent studies have demonstrated that those patients with systolic heart failure who have increased CO_2 chemosensitivity below and above eupnea are prone to develop central apnea during sleep. Obstructive sleep apnea also occurs frequently in patients with heart failure, particularly in those with obesity who presumably have alterations in the mechanical properties of the upper airway. This article reviews the mechanisms of central sleep apnea, obstructive sleep apnea, and periodic breathing in systolic heart failure.

There are no guidelines for the treatment of sleep apnea in heart failure. Central sleep apnea remains difficult to treat and well designed, long-term controlled studies are needed to determine if any treatment prolongs survival. However, based on the pathophysiologic consequences of sleep apnea on the cardiovascular system, studies associating excess mortality of heart failure patients with obstructive and central sleep apnea, and limited favorable therapeutic studies, it is important to continue to identify heart failure patients who may suffer from sleep apnea and treat them appropriately.

ELSEVIER
SAUNDERS

SLEEP
MEDICINE
CLINICS

Sleep Med Clin 2 (2007) xi–xii

Foreword

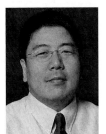

Teofilo Lee-Chiong, Jr., MD
Consulting Editor

Teofilo Lee-Chiong, Jr., MD
Section of Sleep Medicine
National Jewish Medical and Research Center
University of Colorado Health Sciences Center
Denver, CO 80206, USA

E-mail address:
lee-chiongt@njc.org

Significant changes in cardiovascular physiology occur during sleep. Sleep influences cardiovascular physiology primarily by its effect on the autonomic nervous system. Activation of the parasympathetic nervous system during non-rapid eye movement (NREM) sleep gives rise to a reduction in heart rate, cardiac output, and systolic blood pressure compared to levels associated with wakefulness. These changes are magnified further during tonic rapid eye movement (REM) sleep because of sleep-state dependent changes in sympathetic and parasympathetic neural tone, which can result in relative bradycardia and even periods of asystole. Nighttime systolic blood pressure is, therefore, typically less than that during the daytime, a phenomenon referred to as "dipping." In contrast, fluctuating autonomic activity during phasic REM sleep may give rise to transient increases in heart rate, cardiac contractility, and blood pressure because of stimulation of adrenergic alpha-1 receptors. Increases in heart rate and blood pressure also accompany arousals from sleep. Stroke volume and peripheral vascular resistance are minimally affected by sleep. These changes may be responsible, at least in part, for the development of cardiovascular events during sleep, with bradycardia and hypotension responsible for ischemia during NREM sleep, and coronary vasospasm occurring during REM sleep.

Cardiovascular disorders can, in turn, alter sleep architecture and cause disturbances of sleep. The interaction between sleep and cardiovascular disorders is best characterized among patients with obstructive sleep apnea (OSA).

Obstructive sleep apnea is a risk factor for hypertension, with the prevalence and degree of blood pressure elevation correlating significantly with increasing severity of measures of sleep-related breathing disorder, such as apnea-hypopnea index and nocturnal oxygen desaturation. The "dipping" phenomena may be lost in patients with obstructive sleep apnea. This relationship between hypertension and OSA may be particularly relevant in cases of therapy-resistant hypertension. A reduction in blood pressure has been described in some studies during optimal positive airway pressure therapy for OSA.

In middle-aged patients with OSA, the risk of ischemic heart disease (including myocardial infarction, angina, and coronary revascularization procedures) is also increased independent of age,

1556-407X/07/$ – see front matter © 2007 Elsevier Inc. All rights reserved.
sleep.theclinics.com

doi:10.1016/j.jsmc.2007.09.002

body mass index, blood pressure, and history of smoking. This risk is reduced by reversal of obstructive sleep apnea. Possible mechanisms responsible for OSA-related atherosclerosis include an increase in sympathetic activity during sleep, development of insulin resistance, endothelial dysfunction, and increases in hypercoagulability, oxidative stress, and inflammation. OSA is associated with elevated levels of proinflammatory cytokines, adhesion molecules, plasma C-reactive protein, plasma fibrinogen, and platelet activity, as well as reduced fibrinolytic capacity.

Sleep has a variable effect on cardiac arrhythmias. The frequency of premature ventricular contractions may diminish during NREM sleep because of greater parasympathetic activity. Alternatively, ventricular arrhythmias may become more frequent during arousals from sleep due to the surge in sympathetic tone. Arrhythmias associated with OSA include sinus arrhythmia, with slowing of heart rate at the onset of respiratory events and relative tachycardia after the end of the event. Other OSA-related rhythm disturbances, including heart blocks, sinus pauses, supraventricular tachycardia, and ventricular tachycardia or fibrillation, appear to be correlated with the severity of sleep disordered breathing.

Both OSA and central sleep apnea (CSA) can develop in patients with congestive heart failure (CHF). Left ventricular systolic dysfunction is an independent risk factor for sleep disordered breathing in those with CHF. The development of CSA in patients with CHF may be related to alterations in control of CO_2 or a decrease in circulation, both of which may significantly influence loop gain. Cheyne-Stokes respiration (CSR), characterized by periodic crescendo and decrescendo breathing pattern with apneas or hypopneas, is also seen in patients with CHF, predominantly during NREM sleep. Increased mortality in patients with CHF who also develop CSR during sleep compared to those without CSR has been reported.

Finally, OSA can increase the risk of cerebrovascular disease, and vice versa. OSA also negatively influences prognosis following strokes.

Clearly, future research will expand our understanding of the bi-directional relationship between sleep and cardiovascular disorders. Particularly relevant is the potential impact of therapy of OSA on the prevention and management of hypertension, ischemic heart disease, congestive heart failure, and stroke.

SLEEP
MEDICINE
CLINICS

Sleep Med Clin 2 (2007) xiii–xiv

Preface

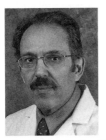

Shahrokh Javaheri, MD
Guest Editor

Shahrokh Javaheri, MD
*Sleepcare Diagnostics 4780 Socialville-Fosters Road
Mason, Ohio 45040*

E-mail address:
javaheri@snorenomore.com

This issue of *Sleep Medicine Clinics* is devoted to cardiovascular disease and sleep-related disorders with an emphasis on sleep apnea. Cardiovascular disorders continue to be highly prevalent and associated with excessive morbidity and mortality and huge economic costs. Updated data indicate that approximately 71 million American adults suffer from one or more types of cardiovascular diseases. Twenty-seven million of these individuals are aged 65 years or older [1]. Meanwhile, sleep-related breathing disorders also are common, particularly in the older population.

Since the early 1900s, cardiovascular disease has been the leading cause of death every year, except in 1918. In 2003, cardiovascular disorders accounted for 37% of all deaths. Each day, 2,500 Americans die from cardiovascular disease—nearly one death every 35 seconds. Approximately 65 million Americans have hypertension, a disorder that has been proven to be associated with obstructive sleep apnea. Approximately 13 million Americans have coronary heart disease, whereas 5 million have heart failure, and 5.5 million have stroke. In the United States and Europe, approximately 15 million individuals have heart failure. The indirect cost of heart failure alone in the United States has been approximately $30 billion [1].

With increasing global adiposity, the prevalence of obstructive sleep apnea is on the rise. The data collected in the late 1980s and published in the early 1990s [1] show a prevalence of Obstructive Sleep Apnea Hypopnea Syndrome in 2% to 4% of the population in the United States. Since then, however, obesity has become an epidemic, and, as a result, the prevalence of sleep apnea has increased considerably. The Wisconsin data [2] underestimate the prevalence of sleep apnea in 2006–2007 [3].

One of the most significant advances in clinical medicine has been the understanding that obstructive sleep apnea could be a cause or contributor to the morbidity or mortality of various cardiovascular disorders. These potential consequences include systemic and pulmonary hypertension and coronary artery disease, including angina, myocardial infarction, heart failure (both systolic and diastolic dysfunction), arrhythmias, and stroke. Conversely, congestive heart failure with left ventricular systolic dysfunction is, perhaps, the most important risk factor for sleep apnea—both obstructive and central sleep apnea.

doi:10.1016/j.jsmc.2007.09.001

Recent studies, which are discussed in this issue, have shown that severe obstructive sleep apnea is associated with excess morbidity and mortality. One study concludes that 45% of subjects with severe obstructive sleep apnea after left untreated, either died or suffered from a significant cardiovascular and cerebrovascular event in the following 10 to 12 years [1]. In contrast, effective treatment of obstructive sleep apnea with CPAP prevents incident cardiovascular and cerebrovascular disease.

Similarly, recent data show that in patients with congestive heart failure, both central and obstructive sleep apnea contribute to mortality, and effective treatment of obstructive and central sleep apnea may improve left ventricular ejection fraction and mortality.

Clearly, more work needs to be done, but we have come a long way in understanding the importance of sleep apnea and its contribution to genesis and/or progression of cardiovascular and cerebrovascular disease.

References

[1] Thom T, Haase N, Rosamond W, et al. Heart disease and stroke statistics—2006 update: a report from the American Heart Association statistics committee and stroke statistics subcommittee. Circulation 2006;113:85–181.

[2] Young T, Palta M, Dempsey J, et al. The occurrence of sleep-disordered breathing among middle-aged adults. N Engl J Med 1993;328:1230–5.

[3] Hiestand D, Britz P, Goldman M, et al. Prevalence of symptoms and risk of sleep apnea in the US population. Chest 2006;130:780–6.

SLEEP
MEDICINE
CLINICS

Sleep Med Clin 2 (2007) 529–538

Cardiovascular Implications of Poor Sleep

Michael H. Bonnet, PhD[a,b,*], Donna L. Arand, PhD[a,b]

- Insomnia and cardiovascular measures
- Insomnia and hypertension
- Insomnia and heart disease
- Sleep deprivation and restriction
- Burnout or vital exhaustion
- Sleep fragmentation
- Summary
- References

A discussion of cardiovascular symptoms secondary to poor sleep would seem to be straightforward at first glance. Unfortunately, poor sleep can have many connotations, and an examination of cardiovascular relationships must be done with reference to the various definitions of poor sleep. The most common connotation of poor sleep is insomnia. Sleep may be less than optimal for a number of additional reasons, however, including lack of opportunity (partial or total sleep deprivation); fragmentation (frequent, repetitive disturbance during sleep); or stress not producing traditional insomnia (burn out or vital exhaustion). Each of these types of poor sleep is discussed. Poor sleep may also be associated with a number of medical disorders, however, such as sleep apnea, Parkinson's disease, or fibromyalgia, but the relationship of medical disorders that produce insomnia to cardiovascular disease is not discussed in this article.

Insomnia and cardiovascular measures

Insomnia is typically defined as difficulty initiating or maintaining sleep with a secondary complaint of compromised daytime function, such as subjective fatigue or perceived inability to perform optimally. Numerous studies have examined sleep and other physiologic variables in patients with primary insomnia and in control populations usually matched with insomnia patients by age, gender, and weight or body mass index (BMI). Both direct cardiac measures and other measures, such as metabolic rate and cortisol, which may have a direct impact on cardiac function have been described. Five controlled studies (including an early study of good and poor sleepers [1]) have been reported. The study of good and poor sleepers documented that poor sleepers had elevated heart rate compared with good sleepers (7 bpm higher 30 minutes before sleep, 6 bpm higher on average during the 30 minutes before sleep, and 4 bpm higher during the sleep period) with both presleep differences being statistically significant. More recent studies [2,3] with insomnia patients and normal control groups identified by complaint and confirmed with polysomnographic recordings have shown that insomnia patients had elevated heart rate throughout the night and in direct sleep stage comparisons.

Supported by the Dayton Department of Veterans Affairs Medical Center, Wright State University School of Medicine, and the Sleep-Wake Disorders Research Institute.
[a] Dayton Department of Veterans Affairs Medical Center, Wright State University School of Medicine, 4100 West Third Street, Dayton, OH 45428, USA
[b] Wallace Kettering Neuroscience Institute, 3533 Southern Boulevard, Suite 5200, Kettering, OH 45429, USA
* Corresponding author. Dayton Department of Veterans Affairs Medical Center, 4100 West Third Street, Dayton, OH 45428.
E-mail address: bonnetmichael@yahoo.com (M.H. Bonnet).

doi:10.1016/j.jsmc.2007.07.007

Stepanski and colleagues [3] found a significantly higher heart rate overall in insomnia patients compared with normals (about 4.4 bpm difference) and a significant consistent increase across wakefulness, non–rapid eye movement sleep, and rapid eye movement sleep (Table 1). Bonnet and Arand [2] found a significant overall effect for heart rate elevation (analyzed from heart period) in insomnia patients compared with normals (about 6.9 bpm difference overall) and a significant consistent increase across wakefulness and sleep stages. The Bonnet and Arand [2] study also analyzed the same 5-minute blocks used for heart rate to calculate heart period spectral parameters. The results were comparable with the heart rate data: the ratio of low-to-high frequency power was significantly greater in insomnia patients both during wake and across sleep stages compared with normals and the ratio of high-frequency to total spectral power was significantly elevated in normal subjects during wake and across sleep stages compared with insomnia patients [2]. Two additional studies that did not report individual sleep stage amounts have also shown elevated heart rate in insomnia patients compared with controls. Haynes and colleagues [4] found a significant 4.6 bpm increase in heart rate in insomnia patients compared with controls in measurements made at sleep onset, and Varkevisser and colleagues [5] reported a nonsignificant 4.1 bpm increase in heart rate in insomnia patients compared with controls in waking measurements made during a constant routine protocol. The nonsignificant finding in the latter study may have been related to the fact that normal baseline sleep was apparently not required for participants in the control group, which had a poor overall sleep efficiency (82%) [6]. Two studies have also looked at heart rate in insomnia patients compared with controls under stressful conditions to test the generality of the heart rate elevation. In one study, insomnia patients had significant and constant elevation in heart rate compared with normal controls throughout a 4-minute stressed

reaction time task [3] given in the morning. Haynes and colleagues [4] reported that their insomnia patients had significantly elevated heart rate before and after but not during a mental arithmetic task presented while the Ss were in bed.

Elevated heart rate in patients with primary insomnia is just one of numerous physiologic differences reported. Other significant differences in these patients include elevated 24-hour whole-body metabolic rate (as measured by VO_2) [7]; elevated brain metabolic rate (positron emission tomography results) [8]; increased cortisol and adrenocorticotropic hormone secretion [9]; increased interleukin-6 [10]; and increased beta electroencephalogram (EEG) activity [11]. Another study has shown that increasingly poor sleep in insomnia patients is correlated with norepinephrine, epinephrine, and dopamine precursors and metabolites [12]. All of these results are consistent with sympathetic or hypothalamic-pituitary-adrenal (HPA) activation. Primary insomnia is frequently a chronic condition [13], and this implies that patients may remain in a sympathetic dominant or HPA-activated state for many years. As such, these patients might be expected to develop cardiovascular problems secondary to the arousal that also produces poor sleep.

Insomnia and hypertension

A number of studies have linked insomnia with the development of hypertension or other cardiac problems. Unfortunately, these studies are almost exclusively questionnaire studies where patients with insomnia are compared with good sleepers and then followed to determine if the incidence of various medical problems increases over time. Studies of long-term treatment or placebo administration in insomnia patients to determine differential outcomes are largely nonexistent.

General health questionnaire studies have typically shown relationships between insomnia, stress, and cardiac variables, such as hypertension [14,15].

Table 1: Heart rate by sleep stage in primary insomnia and controls

Stage	Stepanski et al [3] Heart rate		Bonnet and Arand [2] Heart rate		Bonnet and Arand [2] Low/high power	
	Insomnia	Normal	Insomnia	Normal	Insomnia	Normal
Wake	70.5 (9)	64.5 (7.3)	68.8 (9)	61.7 (7.8)	1.23	0.87
Stage 1			66.0 (9.1)	59.8 (7.9)	1.06	0.80
Stage 2	62.3 (8.6)	59.2 (6.6)	65.6 (9.1)	58.8 (8.7)	0.88	0.64
SWS			68.4 (7.2)	57.9 (6.3)		
REM	64.8 (8.3)	60.9 (8)	68.3 (8.3)	60.4 (8.4)	1.02	0.87

Abbreviations: REM, rapid eye movement; SWS, slow wave sleep.

In one prospective study [16] about 8000 Japanese male middle-age telecommunication workers were classified to have sleep-onset, sleep maintenance insomnia, or normal sleep. Four years later, it was found that 40% of the workers who were identified as having sleep-onset insomnia at the first time point and 42% of the workers who were initially identified as having difficulty staying asleep had developed hypertension, whereas 31% of workers without a sleep problem at the initial time point had developed hypertension (both significant). After adjusting for age, BMI, smoking, alcohol consumption, and job stress, difficulty maintaining sleep was associated with increased hypertension with an odds ratio of 1.88 (95% confidence interval [CI], 1.45–2.45). The authors speculated that this increase in hypertension might be related to activation of the hypothalamic-pituitary-adrenal axis [9,12,17].

Insomnia and heart disease

In a review of epidemiologic studies of the relationship between insomnia and heart disease, Schwartz and colleagues [18] performed a meta-analysis of 10 studies that had examined the relationship between trouble falling asleep and heart disease measures, such as myocardial infarction (MI), and reported a combined risk ratio of 1.92 (95% CI, 1.62–2.31). This result was similar to that found when combining only the four most methodologically strong studies (risk ratio of 1.70 with a 95% CI, 1.33–2.17). In one of the latter studies, from the Framingham study data, Eaker and colleagues [19] analyzed data from 749 women over 20 years and reported a risk ratio of 3.9 for the relationship between trouble falling asleep and MI or coronary heart disease death after adjusting for age, systolic blood pressure, cholesterol, diabetes, smoking, and BMI. In a second strong study [20], the risk ratio for trouble falling asleep with the same cardiac outcome was 1.62 (95% CI, 0.94–2.82) after adjusting for age, cholesterol, blood pressure, and smoking in a group of Scandinavian men. The numerous other results reviewed by Schwartz and colleagues [18] suggested a substantial link between insomnia and cardiovascular outcome. Since that review was published in 1999, several additional studies have appeared. The 10 studies in the Schwartz meta-analysis and six newer studies are summarized in Table 2 [13,14,21–32]. The additional studies since 1999 have continued to show significant links between various definitions of insomnia and general cardiac outcomes. Odds or risk ratios for these studies for the relationship between general insomnia variables and heart disease outcomes ranged from 1.21 to 3.1 and further

enhance the results reported by Schwartz and colleagues [18]. A study by Taylor and colleagues [23] is of note because sleep logs were used to refine the insomnia diagnosis carefully, and several additional questions were asked about snoring, sleep-associated breathing problems, and limb movements or restlessness to adjust for other sleep disorders. Despite adjustment for sleep disorders in addition to depression and anxiety, the odds ratio for the association of insomnia with both heart disease and high blood pressure were still significant (2.27 and 95% CI, 1.13–4.56; 3.18 and 95% CI, 1.90–5.32, respectively). The Nilsson and colleagues [24] study showed that men with poor sleep had an increased odds ratio of cardiac death (1.71). The study also showed that men with an elevated heart rate had an increased risk of cardiac death (odds ratio 1.30) and that men with both poor sleep and a basal heart rate of 71+ bpm had a greatly increased risk of cardiac death (odds ratio 2.66; 95% CI, 2.06–3.44).

As Schwartz and colleagues [18] noted, however, the positive outcomes for odds ratios may occur either because (1) insomnia itself increases the risk of heart disease; (2) insomnia may be only coincidentally associated with heart disease or risk factors for heart disease; or (3) insomnia may be a marker or correlate for other risk factors (eg, depression) that are associated with heart disease.

The most common possible coincidental relationship between insomnia and cardiovascular disease is through the possible relation of insomnia to sleep apnea because of the established link between sleep apnea and cardiac disease [33]. The epidemiologic studies of insomnia and cardiovascular events have all been based on subjective reports of poor sleep, and it is not certain to what extent the outcomes could be based on sleep apnea. It is the case that the most common selection factor, trouble falling asleep, is not a correlate of sleep-associated breathing problems and that insomnia, in general, is not strongly associated with sleep apnea [34,35]. Many authors have also attempted to control for underlying sleep apnea by using reports of snoring or breathing problems at night. Additionally, BMI, a major determiner of sleep apnea, has been controlled in the studies. This criticism will only be completely removed, however, when the degree of sleep apnea itself can be quantified and controlled in these studies.

It is likely that insomnia is a precursor or correlate of other medical problems that are associated with heart disease. For example, insomnia is a strong predictor of later development of depression [36] and a very common symptom of depression. As such, it is possible that an insomnia symptom at one point could predict the development of

Table 2: Studies showing cardiac risk secondary to poor sleep or difficulty falling asleep

Reference	Event	Covariates	Significant effect (poor sleep)	Risk ratio difficulty falling asleep
[25][a]	Combined cardiac	Age	Men: 2.04[c] Women: 2.23[b]	
[20][a]	Combined cardiac	Age, cholesterol, BP, smoker		1.62 (0.94–2.82)
[26][a]	Combined cardiac	None	Men (only) 1.96[b]	
[19][a]	Combined cardiac	Age, BP, BMI, smoke, cholesterol, diabetes		3.9 (1.7–9)
[27][a]	Combined cardiac	Age, gender, health, medicines	1.76 (1.03–3.02)	1.71 (0.86–3.43)
[28][a]	First MI	Age	Increase versus control	
[29][a]	First MI	Match on demographics		Significant increase versus control
[30][a]	First MI	Age, coffee, smoker, type A versus hospital control	1.9 (1.2–3.2)	1.9 (1–3.1)
[31][a]	First MI	Age, gender, BP, smoke, diabetes, cholesterol	Men 2.92 (1.65–5.15)	
[32][a]	First MI	Middle-age men		
[27][a]	First MI	Age, gender, race	1.55 (1.09–2.20)	1.67 (1.08–2.58)
[21]	Combined cardiac	Age, smoke, BMI, depression, snore, medical disease, sleep duration	M but not F	3.1 (1.5–6.3)
[13]	MI	Sociodemographic, health habits	1.6 (1.1–2.7)	
[23]	Heart disease	Depression, anxiety, sleep disorders	2.27 (1.13–4.56)	
[14]	Circulatory disease	Sociodemographic, lifestyle, stress physical	1.21 (1.02–1.43) $P < .01$	
[22]	Heart disease	Age, sex, income, education	1.76 (1.23–2.51)	
[24]	Cardio mortality	Age, BMI, BP, alcohol, cholesterol	M: 1.71 (1.34–2.18) F: 1.67 (0.96–2.90)	M: 1.25 (0.94–1.66) F: 1.93 (1.07–3.47)

Abbreviations: BMI, body mass index; BP, blood pressure; MI, myocardial infarction.
[a] As reviewed in Schwartz et al [18].
[b] $P < .05$.
[c] $P < .01$.

depression, which itself is associated with an increased risk of MI and other cardiac events [37,38]. This argument has been challenged by some recent studies, however, which have controlled for depression and still found insomnia to be related to cardiac events [21,23]. Other medical correlates may exist; however, it is equally likely that other physiologic changes, such as shifting sympathetic-parasympathetic balance, underlie both the development of insomnia and depression.

It is most likely that insomnia itself is highly related to stress where reactivity to stress probably has a genetic and an age component. The implication is that some individuals have a predisposition to sympathetic or HPA activation so that relatively small amounts of situational stress produce both insomnia and an increased cardiovascular risk [2]. Age-related increases in sympathetic activity [39] associated with age-related increases in heart rate compound the effects of life stress and continue to magnify cardiovascular risks.

Sleep deprivation and restriction

Heart rate and blood pressure measures have been reported from sleep deprivation studies for many years. In the older literature, heart rate either did not change or was decreased after total sleep deprivation [40,41]. In one study, Corcoran [40] concluded that heart rate fell with loss of sleep unless subjects needed to expend effort to stay awake, and this effort might be related to lack of change or increase in physiologic measures. More recent sleep deprivation findings have been reviewed by Zhong and colleagues [42]. In a discussion of disparate findings from numerous studies of sleep deprivation, Zhong and colleagues [42] concluded that significant effects on cardiac variables seemed less likely to be reported from studies where measures were made from supine participants and that increases in cardiac measures were more likely to be apparent in studies where measures were made from seated subjects. Eleven studies that have examined heart rate, blood pressure, and other related parameters during and after periods of total sleep deprivation are summarized in Table 3 [40–50]. Of 13 groups in studies reporting heart rate, 9 did not find a significant difference after total sleep loss, 1 found a significant increase, and 3 found a significant decrease. Data were combined from study groups where possible (seven groups) to perform an omnibus *t* test (Table 4) that indicated a nonsignificant 0.5 bpm decrease in heart rate during total sleep deprivation. For systolic and diastolic blood pressure, seven groups were found to have no difference after sleep deprivation, and two groups had significant increases (other studies did not report blood pressure). The combined *t* values from four (systolic) and five (diastolic) groups, however, were both statistically significant in showing increases in blood pressure after total sleep deprivation (see Table 4).

Four studies have reported heart rate or blood pressure changes after 1 night of partial sleep

Table 3: **Studies of cardiac variables during total sleep deprivation, partial sleep deprivation, and sleep restriction**

	Subjects	Position	Heart rate	Systolic pressure	Diastolic pressure	Other
			TSD study			
[42]	18 YA	Supine	Decrease[a]	NS	NS	HRV NS
[42]		Sitting	Increase	NS	NS	HRV NS
[42]		Sitting RT	NS	NS	NS	HRV Sig
[41]	4 YA	Sitting	NS	NS	NS	
[40]	19 YA	Supine	NS	—	—	—
[44]	6 YA	Sitting	NS	—	—	
[43]	8 40-YO	Supine	NS	Increase	Increase	MSNA decrease
[45]	12 YA	Supine	NS	NS	NS	
[46]	15 YA	Sitting	Decrease	—	—	—
[50]	21 YA	—	NS	NS	NS	
[47]	10 YA	—	NS	Increase	NS	CRP increase
[48]	12 YA	Supine	Decrease	—	—	SNS decrease
[49]	6 YA	Supine	NS	NS	Increase	MSNA decrease
			PSD study			
[53]	36 HTN	Sitting	Increase	Increase	Increase	EPI increase
[51]	18 YA, 1 3.6-h sleep	Ambulatory	NS	Increase	Increase	HRV EPI increase
[52]	18 YA, 1 5-h sleep		Increase	Increase	NS	
[54]	36 44-YO	Supine	NS	Increase	Increase	NE EPI NS
[54]	36 alcohol dependent	Supine	Increase	Increase	Increase	NE EPI increase
			Sleep restriction			
[47]	10 YA, 10 4.2-h sleep	—	Increase	NS	NS	CRP increase
[55]	11 YA, 6 4-h sleep	—	—	—	—	HRV sig
[56]	10 60-yr-old F, 3 4-h sleep	—	—	—	—	Cholesterol, LDL increase

Abbreviations: CRP, C-reactive protein; EPI, epinephrine; HRV, heart rate variability; HTN, hypertension; LDL, low-density lipoprotein; MSNA, muscle sympathetic nerve activity; NE, norepinephrine; NS, nonsignificant; PSD, partial sleep deprivation; RT, with performance; SNS, sympathetic activity; TSD, total sleep deprivation; YA, young adult; YO, year-old.
[a] Decrease and Increase refer to corresponding significant changes.

Table 4: Group analysis of cardiac measures

	N	Baseline	Sleep Deprivation	t
Total sleep deprivation				
Heart rate	76	68.5 (4.03)	68.0 (3.78)	−0.999
Systolic blood pressure	36	117.2 (8.8)	122.3 (8.8)	2.459[a]
Diastolic blood pressure	42	63.9 (6.88)	67.2 (6.7)	2.360[a]
Partial sleep deprivation				
Heart rate	126	61.2 (12.97)	67.9 (8.48)	4.855[a]
Systolic blood pressure	126	119.0 (16)	132.1 (7.5)	8.419[a]
Diastolic blood pressure	54	86.9 (7.2)	90.5 (6.8)	2.668[a]

[a] $P < .05$.

deprivation, with sleep time reduced to from 3.6 to 5 hours [51–54]. In the five groups in these studies, heart rate was significantly increased in three, systolic blood pressure was increased in five, and diastolic blood pressure was increased in four. The combined t values for these three measures (see Table 4) were all statistically significant. There is no clear rationale explaining why these differences were much larger than those after 1 night of total sleep deprivation. The studies in this category were the only ones performed in clinical groups (alcohol-dependent patients and patients with diagnosed hypertension), however, and significant findings in those clinical groups accounted for 6 of the 12 significant findings in these studies. It is likely that subjects with increased stress or existing medical problems related to arousal might respond more significantly to stressful sleep deprivation conditions to show increased blood pressure and heart rate.

Three studies of cardiac measures after sleep restriction for 3 to 10 nights were found (see Table 3 for summary) [47,55,56], but only the study by Meier-Ewart and colleagues [47] reported heart rate and blood pressure (finding a significant increase in heart rate but not blood pressure). This study, which involved 10 consecutive nights with 4.2 hours of sleep in normals, was the most arduous restriction study but, compared with the single night restriction studies previously mentioned, did not find significant increases in either measure of blood pressure [47].

Another means of approaching sleep restriction is evaluation of medical outcomes in relation to habitual sleep duration with the assumption that individuals with very short sleep durations are likely to have restricted sleep. In one recent study [57], the relationship between sleep duration and hypertension was examined in data from the National Health and Nutrition Examination Study. In the overall data set, those participants with a normal sleep duration of 5 hours per night or less had a significantly increased odds ratio for hypertension at 8- to 10-year follow-up for unadjusted data and for each of three adjusted models (adjustments included daytime sleepiness, depression, activity, alcohol, salt, smoking, heart rate, and gender; education, age, and ethnicity; and BMI and diabetes). The study also found that all of these relationships were stronger in younger participants (age, 32–59 years) and nonsignificant in older participants (age, 60–86 years). Results for 6-hour sleepers were not significant. In a large study of nurses [58], it was found that short sleep times of 5 or fewer hours per night were not significantly associated with cardiovascular death (odds ratio, 1.04; 95% CI, 0.79–1.35). Similarly, Wingard and Berkman [59] were unable to show a significant association between sleep duration of 6 hours and less and incidence of either ischemic heart disease or stroke. In a final recent study [60], a significant association between sleep duration of less than 5 hours and blood pressure and blood lipids was reported in data from a large sample (40–45 years of age) at a single time point. None of these relationships remained significant, however, after controlling for gender, smoking, and BMI.

Burnout or vital exhaustion

Patients identified by their subjective reports of excess daytime fatigue, loss of vigor, irritability, and demoralization that seem to occur for some months before an MI have been given the label "vital exhaustion." Burnout is an allied concept that is defined broadly as "a state of vital exhaustion," although it is usually in reference to long-term work stress overload. All of these patients suffered from chronic, unremitting stress and sometimes vaguely described poor sleep. An initial population study in Germany [61] found that vital exhaustion was significantly related to MI by the use of logistic regression that controlled for blood pressure, snoring, cholesterol, age, and antihypertensive medication. The effect for fatigue was not as large as that for age, smoking, or cholesterol but was larger than the effect for systolic blood pressure. In a further analysis of individual questionnaire items relating to MI, only 1 of 10 significant items was specifically related to sleep ("do you often have trouble falling asleep?") but the most significant relationship was with waking up with the feeling of exhaustion [62]. In a follow-up study, 17 patients identified as suffering from vital exhaustion or controls had sleep evaluations. More than 55% of the patients with exhaustion reported subjective problems with their sleep (versus none of the control patients), but EEG sleep parameters in the two groups were remarkably similar. The only significant difference was a reduction in slow wave sleep in the exhausted patients (although the difference in delta power was not significant). In a more recent study of burnout [63], matched groups of 12 individuals with high and low burnout scores were compared on numerous measures including polysomnography. The groups did not differ on any objective sleep measures (slow wave sleep was actually nonsignificantly higher in the high burnout patients) except that EEG arousals and arousal index were elevated in the burnout group. As expected, the patients with burnout did complain of insufficient sleep, daytime sleepiness, and impairment at awakening resulting in dissatisfaction with their work performance. In other analyses, the high burnout group was also found to report significantly higher anxiety and depression, while reporting no difference in their overall sleep deficit. In a second publication from this dataset [64], the relationship of elevated EEG arousals was examined in more detail. A stepwise multiple regression analysis showed that number of EEG arousals was the only significant predictor for higher blood pressure (both systolic and diastolic); plasma cortisol at awakening; total cholesterol; and low-density lipoprotein. EEG arousals were also significantly related to salivary cortisol at awakening, heart rate, and low-density/high-density lipoprotein ratio. In simple t test comparisons, those with high arousals had significantly elevated heart rate, diastolic blood pressure, salivary cortisol, total cholesterol, and low-density lipoprotein. The authors speculated that the elevated cardiovascular measures were related to elevated arousals, rather than underlying depression or anxiety, because depression and anxiety scores were added to the multiple regression equations but did not add to the results.

Sleep fragmentation

Sleep fragmentation, most commonly defined as frequent brief arousal from sleep, is a core finding in sleep apnea. Sleep apnea has a large cardiovascular impact, but it is normally believed that the impact is directly related to an obstructed airway and the struggle to breathe. It is less obvious but possible that there is additional cardiac impact from the frequent disturbance of sleep itself. Several studies of empiric sleep fragmentation (ie, EEG disturbance usually by tones with no relationship to respiration) in normal young adults have shown evidence of physiologic activation. Even brief EEG arousals during sleep are associated with increases in heart rate of 9 to 13 bpm lasting 10 to 15 seconds [65] and blood pressure increases that are about 75% of the increase seen after periods of sleep apnea [66]. During an undisturbed night of sleep, heart rate typically decreases by about 12 bpm [67], so that changes associated with brief arousals return heart rate to approximate waking levels. A study of VO_2 during empiric sleep fragmentation in normal young adults [68] showed a significant increase in VO_2 in the 3-minute average following 2- to 5-second EEG arousals and a significant increase in VO_2 for 6 to 9 minutes after longer EEG arousals (15–75 seconds). This means that when brief EEG arousals were produced after each minute of sleep, VO_2 remained elevated to about 95% of presleep waking VO_2 throughout the night. A similar fragmented sleep pattern has also been associated with alteration in plasma cortisol and adrenocorticotropic hormone secretion that is similar to that seen after total sleep deprivation [69].

Only a few clinical studies have examined the relationship of simple sleep fragmentation with cardiovascular variables. One study of individuals with a respiratory disturbance index of less than one found a significant correlation between blood pressure and a sleep fragmentation measure [70]. The burnout studies reviewed in the previous section that demonstrated relationships between EEG arousals and cardiac measures could be an example of either job stress producing EEG arousals and cardiac changes or of an interrelation between stress and EEG arousals to produce cardiac changes. A case study has also reported increases in blood pressure associated with periodic limb movements [71]. These studies suggest that many conditions that can produce frequent sleep disturbance without relation to specific respiratory problems can also produce chronic elevation in cardiovascular measures. Much work remains to determine whether such chronic disturbance may also be related to important cardiovascular consequences.

Summary

Sleep may be degraded in numerous ways by genetic disposition, lifestyle choice, aging, or learned habits. In general, deficits related to a single night of poor or reduced sleep are reversed in the next sleep period. Chronic shortening or disruption of sleep, however, seems to be both a result and cause of physiologic arousal. The components of chronic arousal can be genetic or learned. Such arousal may be one underlying cause of insomnia, psychiatric disorders, and, eventually, cardiac disease. When such arousal produces insomnia, the reduced sleep and stress that becomes associated with sleep may feed back to intensify the underlying arousal or promote a situational problem to a chronic one. Stress, associated with an overcommitted lifestyle, can produce chronic sleep restriction that may also feed back to increase arousal. Finally, decreases in activity that accompany aging can produce a shift to sympathetic dominance that may both produce insomnia and increase cardiac risk factors. It is not surprising that reduced or disturbed sleep may contribute to cardiac dysfunction. The challenge for the future is to determine if treatment (normalization of sleep times, use of hypnotics or behavioral therapy for insomnia, reduction of stress) can produce normalization of cardiac measures and decreased mortality.

References

[1] Monroe LJ. Psychological and physiological differences between good and poor sleepers. J Abnorm Psychol 1967;72:255–64.

[2] Bonnet MH, Arand DL. Heart rate variability in insomniacs and matched normal sleepers. Psychosom Med 1998;60:610–5.

[3] Stepanski E, Glinn M, Zorick FJ, et al. Heart rate changes in chronic insomnia. Stress Med 1994; 10:261–6.

[4] Haynes SN, Adams A, Franzen M. The effects of presleep stress on sleep-onset insomnia. J Abnorm Psychol 1981;90:601–6.

[5] Varkevisser M, Van Dongen HP, Kerkhof GA. Physiologic indexes in chronic insomnia during a constant routine: evidence for general hyperarousal? Sleep 2005;28:1588–96.

[6] Bonnet MH. Hyperarousal as the basis for insomnia: effect size and significance. Sleep 2005; 28:1214–5.

[7] Bonnet MH, Arand DL. 24-hour metabolic rate in insomniacs and matched normal sleepers. Sleep 1995;18:581–8.

[8] Nofzinger EA, Buysse DJ, Germain A, et al. Insomnia: functional neuroimaging evidence for hyperarousal. Am J Psychiatry 2004;161:2126–8.

[9] Vgontzas AN, Bixler EO, Lin H, et al. Chronic insomnia is associated with nyctohemeral activation of the hypothalamic-pituitary axis: clinical implications. J Clin Endocrinol Metab 2001;86: 3787–94.

[10] Burgos I, Richter L, Klein T, et al. Increased nocturnal interleukin-6 excretion in patients with primary insomnia: a pilot study. Brain Behav Immun 2006;20:246–53.

[11] Perlis ML, Merica H, Smith MT, et al. Beta EEG activity and insomnia. Sleep Med Rev 2001;5: 363–74.

[12] Vgontzas AN, Tsigos C, Bixler EO, et al. Chronic insomnia and activity of the stress system: a preliminary study. J Psychosom Res 1998;45:21–31.

[13] Katz DA, McHorney CA. Clinical correlates of insomnia in patients with chronic illness. Arch Intern Med 1998;158:1099–107.

[14] Sutton DA, Moldofsky H, Bradley EM. Insomnia and health problems in Canadians. Sleep 2001; 24:665–70.

[15] Gislason T, Almqvist M. Somatic diseases and sleep complaints: an epidemiological study of 3,201 Swedish men. Acta Med Scand 1987;221: 475–81.

[16] Suka M, Yoshida K, Sugimori H. Persistent insomnia is a predictor of hypertension in Japanese male workers. J Occup Health 2003;45: 344–50.

[17] Rodenbeck A, Hajak G. Neuroendocrine dysregulation in primary insomnia. Rev Neurol 2001;157:5S57–61.

[18] Schwartz S, Anderson WM, Cole SR, et al. Insomnia and heart disease: a review of epidemiologic studies. J Psychosom Res 1999;47:313–33.

[19] Eaker ED, Pinsky J, Castelli WP. Myocardial infarction and coronary death among women: psychosocial predictors from a 20-year follow-up of women in the Framingham Study. Am J Epidemiol 1992;135:854–64.

[20] Appels A, de Vos Y, van Diest R, et al. Are sleep complaints predictive of future myocardial infarction? Act Nerv Super (Praha) 1987;29: 147–51.

[21] Mallon L, Broman JE, Hetta J. Sleep complaints predict coronary artery disease mortality in males: a 12-year follow-up study of a middle-aged Swedish population. J Intern Med 2002; 251:207–16.

[22] Foley DJ, Monjan A, Simonsick EM, et al. Incidence and remission of insomnia among elderly adults: an epidemiologic study of 6,800 persons over three years. Sleep 1999;22(Suppl 2): S366–72.

[23] Taylor DJ, Mallory LJ, Lichstein KL, et al. Comorbidity of chronic insomnia with medical problems. Sleep 2007;30:213–8.

[24] Nilsson PM, Nilsson JA, Hedblad B, et al. Sleep disturbance in association with elevated pulse rate for prediction of mortality: consequences of mental strain? J Intern Med 2001;250:521–9.

[25] Koskenvue M, Kaprio J, Partinen M, et al. Poor sleep quality, emotional stress and morbidity: a six year followup of 10788 persons aged 35–59 years. In: Achte K, Pakaslahti A, editors. Stress and psychosomatics. Helsinki (Finland): Psychiatria Fennica; 1986. p. 115–20.

[26] Siegrist J, Peter R, Motz W. The role of hypertension, left ventricular hypertrophy and

psychosocial risks in cardiovascular disease: prospective evidence from blue-collar men. Eur Heart J 1992;13(Suppl):89–95.

[27] Schwartz S, Cornoni-Huntley J, Cole S, et al. Are sleep complaints an independent risk factor for myocardial infarction? Ann Epidemiol 1998;8:384–92.

[28] Thiel HG, Parker D, Bruce TA. Stress factors and the risk of myocardial infarction. J Psychosom Res 1973;17:43–57.

[29] Friedman GD, Ury HK, Klatsky AL, et al. A psychological questionnaire predictive of myocardial infarction: results from the Kaiser-Permanente epidemiologic study of myocardial infarction. Psychosom Med 1974;36:327–43.

[30] Falgar P, Schouten E, Appels A. Sleep complaints, behavioral characteristics and vital exhaustion in myocardial infarction cases. Psychol Health 1988;2:231–58.

[31] Welin CL, Rosengren A, Wilhelmsen LW. Behavioral characteristics in patients with myocardial infarction: a case-control study. J Cardiovasc Risk 1995;2:247–54.

[32] Vanhalla K. Psychological risk factors related to coronary heart disease. In: Achte KA, editor. Monographs of Psychiatria Fennica. Kyriiri (Finland): Arkadiankatu; 1979.

[33] Wolf J, Lewicka J, Narkiewicz K. Obstructive sleep apnea: an update on mechanisms and cardiovascular consequences. Nutr Metab Cardiovasc Dis 2007;17:233–40.

[34] Roehrs T, Conway W, Wittig R, et al. Sleep-wake complaints in patients with sleep-related respiratory disturbances. Am Rev Respir Dis 1985;132:520–3.

[35] Dickel MJ, Mosko SS. Morbidity cut-offs for sleep apnea and periodic leg movements in predicting subjective complaints in seniors. Sleep 1990;13:155–66.

[36] Breslau N, Roth T, Resenthal L, et al. Sleep disturbance and psychiatric disorders: a longitudinal epidemiological study of young adults. Biol Psychiatry 1996;39:411–8.

[37] Rabins PV, Harvis K, Koven S. High fatality rates of late life depression associated with cardiovascular disease. J Affect Disord 1985;9:165–7.

[38] Carney RM, Freedland KE, Jaffe AS. Insomnia and depression prior to myocardial infarction. Psychosom Med 1990;52:603–9.

[39] Jennings JR, Mack ME. Does aging differentially reduce heart rate variability related to respiration? Exp Aging Res 1984;10:19–23.

[40] Corcoran DW. Changes in heart rate and performance as a result of loss of sleep. Br J Psychol 1964;55:307–14.

[41] Kollar EJ, Pasnau RO, Rubin RT, et al. Psychological, psychophysiological, and biochemical correlates of prolonged sleep deprivation. Am J Psychiatry 1969;126:488–97.

[42] Zhong X, Hilton HJ, Gates GJ, et al. Increased sympathetic and decreased parasympathetic cardiovascular modulation in normal humans with acute sleep deprivation. J Appl Physiol 2005;98:2024–32.

[43] Kato M, Phillips BG, Sigurdsson G, et al. Effects of sleep deprivation on neural circulatory control. Hypertension 2000;35:1173–5.

[44] Fiorica V, Higgins EA, Iampietro PF, et al. Physiological responses of men during sleep deprivation. J Appl Physiol 1968;24:167–76.

[45] Ahnve S, Theorell T, Akerstedt T, et al. Circadian variations in cardiovascular parameters during sleep deprivation: a noninvasive study of young healthy men. Eur J Appl Physiol Occup Physiol 1981;46:9–19.

[46] Chen HI. Effects of 30-h sleep loss on cardiorespiratory functions at rest and in exercise. Med Sci Sports Exerc 1991;23:193–8.

[47] Meier-Ewert HK, Ridker PM, Rifai N, et al. Effect of sleep loss on C-reactive protein, an inflammatory marker of cardiovascular risk. J Am Coll Cardiol 2004;43:678–83.

[48] Holmes AL, Burgess HJ, Dawson D. Effects of sleep pressure on endogenous cardiac autonomic activity and body temperature. J Appl Physiol 2002;92:2578–84.

[49] Ogawa Y, Kanbayashi T, Saito Y, et al. Total sleep deprivation elevates blood pressure through arterial baroreflex resetting: a study with microneurographic technique. Sleep 2003;26:986–9.

[50] Smith A, Maben A. Effects of sleep deprivation, lunch, and personality on performance, mood, and cardiovascular function. Physiol Behav 1993;54:967–72.

[51] Tochikubo O, Ikeda A, Miyajima E, et al. Effects of insufficient sleep on blood pressure monitored by a new multibiomedical recorder. Hypertension 1996;27:1318–24.

[52] Lusardi P, Mugellini A, Preti P, et al. Effects of a restricted sleep regimen on ambulatory blood pressure monitoring in normotensive subjects. Am J Hypertens 1996;9:503–5.

[53] Lusardi P, Zoppi A, Preti P, et al. Effects of insufficient sleep on blood pressure in hypertensive patients: a 24-h study. Am J Hypertens 1999;12:63–8.

[54] Irwin MR, Ziegler M. Sleep deprivation potentiates activation of cardiovascular and catecholamine responses in abstinent alcoholics. Hypertension 2005;45:252–7.

[55] Spiegel K, Leproult R, Van Cauter E. Impact of sleep debt on metabolic and endocrine function. Lancet 1999;354:1435–9.

[56] Kerkhofs M, Boudjeltia KZ, Stenuit P, et al. Sleep restriction increases blood neutrophils, total cholesterol and low density lipoprotein cholesterol in postmenopausal women: a preliminary study. Maturitas 2006;56:212–5.

[57] Gangwisch JE, Heymsfield SB, Boden-Albala B, et al. Short sleep duration as a risk factor for hypertension: analyses of the first National Health and Nutrition Examination Survey. Hypertension 2006;47:833–9.

[58] Patel SR, Ayas NT, Malhotra MR, et al. A prospective study of sleep duration and mortality risk in women. Sleep 2004;27:440–4.

[59] Wingard DL, Berkman LF. Mortality risk associated with sleeping patterns among adults. Sleep 1983;6:102–7.

[60] Bjorvatn B, Sagen IM, Oyane N, et al. The association between sleep duration, body mass index and metabolic measures in the Hordaland Health Study. J Sleep Res 2007;16:66–76.

[61] Appels A, Mulder P. Excess fatigue as a precursor of myocardial infarction. Eur Heart J 1988;9:758–64.

[62] Appels A, Schouten E. Waking up exhausted as risk indicator for myocardial infarction. Am J Cardiol 1991;68:395–8.

[63] Solderstrom M, Ekstedt M, Akerstedt T, et al. Sleep and sleepiness in young individuals with high burnout scores. Sleep 2004;27:1369–77.

[64] Ekstedt M, Akerstedt T, Soderstrom M. Microarousals during sleep are associated with increased levels of lipids, cortisol, and blood pressure. Psychosom Med 2004;66:925–31.

[65] Nalivaiko E, Catcheside PG, Adams A, et al. Cardiac changes during arousals from non-REM sleep in healthy volunteers. Am J Physiol Regul Integr Comp Physiol 2007;292:R1320–7.

[66] Davies RJ, Belt PJ, Roberts SJ, et al. Arterial blood pressure responses to graded transient arousal from sleep in normal humans. J Appl Physiol 1993;74:1123–30.

[67] Viola AU, Simon C, Ehrhart J, et al. Sleep processes exert a predominant influence on the 24-h profile of heart rate variability. J Biol Rhythms 2002;17:539–47.

[68] Bonnet MH, Berry RB, Arand DL. Metabolism during normal sleep, fragmented sleep, and recovery sleep. J Appl Physiol 1991;71:1112–8.

[69] Spath-Schwalbe E, Gofferje M, Kern W, et al. Sleep disruption alters nocturnal ACTH and cortisol secretory patterns. Biol Psychiatry 1991;29:575–84.

[70] Morrell MJ, Finn L, Kim H, et al. Sleep fragmentation, awake blood pressure, and sleep-disordered breathing in a population-based study. Am J Respir Crit Care Med 2000;162:2091–6.

[71] Ali NJ, Davies RJ, Fleetham JA, et al. Periodic movements of the legs during sleep associated with rises in systemic blood pressure. Sleep 1991;14:163–5.

ELSEVIER
SAUNDERS

SLEEP
MEDICINE
CLINICS

Sleep Med Clin 2 (2007) 539–547

Pathophysiologic Mechanisms of Cardiovascular Disease in Obstructive Sleep Apnea

Walter T. McNicholas, MD, FRCPI, FRCPC[a,b,*], Shahrokh Javaheri, MD[c]

- Pathophysiologic sequelae of OSA
  Sympathetic nervous system overactivity
  Inflammation
  Oxidative stress
  Endothelial dysfunction

- *Blood coagulation abnormalities*
  Metabolic dysregulation
  Glucose intolerance
  The leptin pathway
- References

Obstructive sleep apnea (OSA) is a form of periodic breathing characterized by periodic episodes of complete (obstructive apnea) or incomplete (obstructive hypopnea) upper airway occlusion. This sleep breathing disorder is thought to contribute to, or be a cause of systemic and pulmonary hypertension, atherosclerosis, coronary artery disease, heart failure, atrial fibrillation, and stroke. The mechanisms underlying cardiovascular disease in patients with OSA are still poorly understood. The pathogenesis is likely to be a multifactorial process involving a diverse range of mechanisms, including sympathetic nervous system overactivity, selective activation of inflammatory pathways, endothelial dysfunction, and metabolic dysregulation, the latter particularly involving insulin resistance and disordered lipid metabolism.

Pathophysiologic sequelae of OSA

There are three immediate adverse sequelae of OSA [1,2]. These include (1) intermittent arterial blood gas abnormalities, characterized by hypoxemia-reoxygenation and hypercapnia-hypocapnia, (2) arousals, and (3) large negative swings in intrathoracic pressure. These immediate nocturnal consequences of sleep apnea initiate and eventually result in activation of neurohormones, hypercoagulapathy, oxidative stress, release of inflammatory mediators, and increased expression of cellular adhesion molecules, and eventually contribute to structural alterations and remodeling of the cardiac chambers.

Hypoxemia and hypercapnia result in increased sympathetic activity and pulmonary arterial vasoconstriction. Hypoxemia may result in decreased myocardial oxygen delivery, and both hypoxemia and hypoxemia-reoxygenation result in increased expression of redox-sensitive genes, encoding inflammatory mediators such as endothelin [1,2]. These adverse effects of altered blood chemistry may be more deleterious to the cardiovascular system in the setting of pre-existing cardiovascular disease than when the heart is otherwise normal.

The second immediate consequence of sleep apneas and hypopneas is arousal. With each

[a] Respiratory Sleep Disorders Unit, St. Vincent's University Hospital, Elm Park, Dublin 4, Ireland
[b] The Conway Institute of Biomolecular and Biomedical Research, University College, Dublin, Ireland
[c] Sleepcare Diagnostics, 4780 Socialville-Fosters Road, Mason, OH 45040, USA
* Respiratory Sleep Disorders Unit, St. Vincent's University Hospital, Elm Park, Dublin 4, Ireland.
E-mail address: walter.mcnicholas@ucd.ie (W.T. McNicholas).

1556-407X/07/$ – see front matter © 2007 Elsevier Inc. All rights reserved.
doi:10.1016/j.jsmc.2007.08.003
sleep.theclinics.com

arousal, there is transient reinstitution of the wakefulness, increased sympathetic, [3] and decreased parasympathetic activity. Consequently, heart rate and blood pressure increase, resulting in increased myocardial oxygen consumption and afterload, respectively. Arousal-induced sympathetic activity (along with that caused by hypoxemia and hypercapnia) should have acute and deleterious cardiovascular effects, particularly in the setting of heart failure.

Finally, large intrathoracic pressure swings, which occur during obstructive sleep apnea, are reflected in juxtacardiac pressure swings increasing the transmural left ventricular pressure and its wall tension [1,2]. The increase in left ventricular afterload increases myocardial oxygen consumption, may contribute to remodeling of cardiac chambers, and may also cause development of atrial fibrillation (by increasing left atrial transmural pressure). The increase in afterload is particularly deleterious in the setting of left ventricular systolic dysfunction, because the failed left ventricle is very sensitive to small increases in the left ventricular afterload. Finally, increased negative intrathoracic pressure is also transmitted to pulmonary interstitial tissue, and the negative interstitial pressure may contribute to development of pulmonary edema. The remainder of this article examines several intermediary mechanisms of OSA-induced cardiovascular disorders.

While OSA is associated with a diverse range of pathophysiologic features ranging from sleep fragmentation and daytime sleepiness to recurring episodes of apnea-associated oxygen desaturation, there is growing evidence that intermittent hypoxia is a key feature in the cardiovascular pathophysiology of the disorder because of the associated intermittent reoxygenation. This latter feature has been compared with reperfusion injury [1]. A summary of proposed mechanisms of cardiovascular disease in OSA is given in Fig. 1.

Sympathetic nervous system overactivity

The repetitive episodes of upper airway obstruction that are characteristic of OSA result in intermittent hypoxia and large swings in intrathoracic pressure that trigger autonomic responses, including sympathetic nervous system overactivity. Such overactivity has been suggested for many years as playing a role in the pathogenesis of cardiovascular complications in OSA. The theory is based on early reports that found increased urinary catecholamine levels in patients with OSA; these levels fell after treatment by tracheostomy [2]. Another report found a significant fall in both plasma and urinary catecholamines with nasal continuous positive airway pressure (CPAP) in comparison to sham CPAP [4].

A direct link between hypoxemia and elevated sympathetic activity has also been proposed [3,5,6], and elevated muscle sympathetic nerve activity (MSNA) was attenuated during apnea when hyperoxic conditions were maintained [6]. Furthermore, Narkiewicz and colleagues [7] have demonstrated a selective potentiation of peripheral chemoreflex sensitivity in patients with OSA

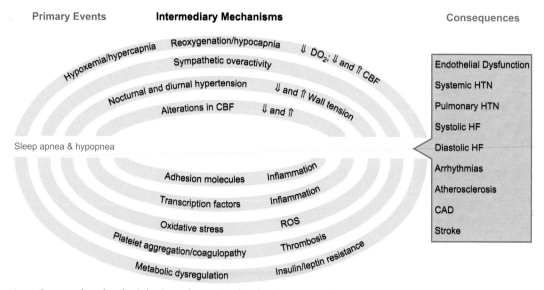

Fig. 1. Proposed pathophysiologic pathways in the development of cardiovascular disease in obstructive sleep apnea. CAD, coronary artery disease; CBF, cerebral/coronary blood flow; $\dot{D}O_2$, oxygen delivery; ⇓, decrease; ⇑, increase; HF, heart failure; HTN, hypertension; ROS, reactive oxygen species. (*Adapted from* Javaheri S. Heart failure and sleep apnea: emphasis on practical therapeutic options. Clin Chest Med 2003;24:211; with permission.)

compared with normal controls. Muscle sympathetic nerve activity has also been directly measured by a tungsten microelectrode inserted into the peroneal nerve. Using this methodology, an increase in MSNA following an acute apnea associated with hypoxia has been observed [8], together with positive correlations between MSNA and plasma norepinephrine levels [9,10]. Treatment with nasal CPAP significantly lowered MSNA [11].

Furthermore, evidence in favor of a significant contribution to the pathogenesis of OSA-related cardiovascular complications, by alterations in autonomic cardiovascular control, has been obtained by techniques exploring spontaneous sensitivity of baroreflex control of the heart [12,13]. OSA patients are characterized by a reduced baroreflex sensitivity during both wakefulness and sleep [14], and such an impairment can be reversed by CPAP. This improvement is particularly evident with chronic treatment [15], although a small but significant improvement can also be detected even after short-term CPAP application [16]. A recent report indicates that intermittent hypoxia is the principal determinant of reduced baroreflex sensitivity in OSA [17].

Support for the role of sympathetic overactivity in the pathogenesis of hypertension in OSA also comes from animal models. An increase in blood pressure was found in both dog and rat models of OSA, which declined once the airway occlusion was abolished [18,19]. These blood pressure changes were not observed with recurrent induced arousals without airway occlusion, indicating that it was the obstructive events rather than the associated arousals that were responsible for the observed effects [18]. These changes in blood pressure were prevented by pharmacologic and surgical blockade of the sympathetic nerve system in a rat model of chronic intermittent hypoxia [20,21].

Inflammation

The role of inflammation in the development of atherosclerosis is well established. Following activation by various stimuli, such as low-density lipoprotein-cholesterol, injury, or infection, inflammatory cells such as macrophages and lymphocytes release cytokines, chemokines, and growth factors [22]. Various markers of inflammation are recognized cardiovascular risk factors, such as the proinflammatory cytokines tumor necrosis factor alpha (TNF-α) and interleukin 6 (IL-6), chemokines such as interleukin 8 (IL-8), adhesion molecules such as soluble intercellular adhesion molecule 1 (ICAM-1), and the acute-phase factor C-reactive protein (CRP) [22,23]. The proinflammatory cytokine TNF-α is an important factor in this process, inducing the expression of cellular adhesion molecules, which mediate adhesion of leucocytes to the vascular endothelium [24,25]. TNF-α is regulated by the transcription factor NFκ-B, a master regulator of inflammatory gene expression [26].

Circulating levels of TNF-α have been shown to correlate with signs of early atherosclerosis amongst healthy middle-aged men [27] and are predictive of coronary heart disease and congestive cardiac failure [28]. Moreover, persistent increased levels of TNF-α after myocardial infarction are predictive of future coronary events [29]. Several studies have identified increased TNF-α levels in OSA patients, and both T-cells and monocytes have been suggested as potential sources [30–33]. Furthermore, a gene polymorphism associated with increased TNF-α production has recently been reported to be more common in OSA [34]. TNF-α levels have also been reported to fall significantly with CPAP therapy [33]. Levels of circulating soluble adhesion molecules, which mediate adhesion of leucocytes to the vascular endothelium, such as ICAM-1, are elevated in patients with OSA and improve with CPAP therapy [35]. Furthermore, increased adhesion of lymphocytes to vascular endothelial cells has been demonstrated in OSA patients compared with controls [31].

The association of CRP with OSA is less clear-cut. CRP is an important serum marker of inflammation, is synthesized in the liver, and regulated by cytokines, particularly IL-6 [36]. CRP is a strong predictor of future coronary events in apparently healthy women [37], in addition to peripheral arterial disease [38]. OSA is reported to be associated with higher CRP and IL-6 levels in otherwise healthy subjects, and these levels correlate with OSA severity [39–42]. Furthermore, treatment with nasal CPAP has been reported to be associated with decreased levels of these markers [40]. However, some recent studies have failed to find an association between CRP and OSA independent of obesity, and the relationship is now less clear-cut [43–45].

Recent evidence from a cell culture model of intermittent hypoxia supports a selective activation of inflammatory, over adaptive, pathways in response to intermittent hypoxia, which contrasts with sustained hypoxia where activation of adaptive and protective pathways predominate [46]. This preferential activation of inflammatory pathways may be a consequence of the intermittent reoxygenation that is characteristic of intermittent hypoxia, and thus represents a variant of reperfusion injury [2]. The activation of inflammatory transcription factors by intermittent hypoxia reoxygenation (IHR) has also been demonstrated in a rat model, where the investigators found a significant correlation with the degree of IHR and neurocognitive function, and also an improvement with reversal of IHR [47].

Hypoxia also induces the activation of the adaptive pathway mediated by up-regulation of the transcription factor hypoxia-inducible factor-1 (HIF-1). There is evidence of HIF-1 dependent gene activation in OSA, as indicated by increased levels of vascular endothelial growth factor [48], although another study indicates that OSA associated with pure intermittent hypoxia (where interapnea oxygen levels are normal) is not associated with elevated levels of another HIF-1 dependent gene, erythropoietin [46].

Oxidative stress

While there is evidence of increased release of reactive oxygen species in patients with OSA [49,50], likely as a consequence of intermittent reoxygenation associated with recurring apnea, the interaction with other molecular mechanisms, such as inflammatory pathways, has not been fully evaluated. Studies in rats demonstrate that chronic intermittent hypoxia (CIH) results in oxidative stress that subsequently leads to left ventricular dysfunction [51]. Similarly, CIH-associated oxidative stress has been shown to result in cortical neuronal cell apoptosis in mice [52]. The oxidative stress-induced brain injury appears to be associated with hypersomnolence in a mouse model of CIH [53,54]. Oxidative stress may be responsible for reduced nitric oxide (NO) bioavailability, enhanced lipid peroxidation [55], and formation of isoprostanes [56], although there is recent evidence that CIH is associated with activation of inducible nitric oxide synthase in the brain [57]. CIH has also been associated with reduced hypoglossal nerve output by oxidative stress [58]. Furthermore, free radicals might up-regulate transcription factors such as NFκ-B and HIF [2].

Endothelial dysfunction

The vascular endothelium controls various vascular functions through regulation of vasoactive mediators in response to physical or biochemical stimuli, and is the major regulator of vascular hemostasis. The endothelium maintains the balance between vasodilatation and vasoconstriction and if this balance is tilted toward vasoconstriction, endothelial dysfunction occurs, causing damage to the arterial wall. Endothelial dysfunction has been found to occur in response to cardiovascular risk factors and to precede or accelerate the development of atherosclerosis [59]. Such dysfunction appears to have a predictive value for cardiovascular events in patients with chest pain or coronary artery disease [60]. Endothelial dysfunction has also been shown to occur in OSA patients with little evidence of cardiovascular disease, and in human studies that assessed intima-media thickness and carotid-

femoral pulse wave velocity [61]. A role for this dysfunction in the pathogenesis of cardiovascular complications in OSA has been supported by various studies demonstrating impairment in endothelium-dependent vasodilatation [62–66]. Furthermore, treatment with nasal CPAP has been reported to reverse endothelial dysfunction [67]. There appears to be a gender difference in endothelial function in that flow-mediated vasodilation is more impaired in females with OSA than males [68].

A major vasodilator substance released by the endothelium is nitric oxide [69] and decreased production or activity of NO may be an early sign of atherosclerosis. Decreased levels of NO have been found in OSA patients and levels increase with CPAP therapy [57,70–74]. The endothelium also produces vasoconstrictor substances, such as endothelin and angiotensin II, and levels have been reported as increased in OSA but to fall with effective CPAP therapy [75]. However, other reports did not find an increase of endothelin in OSA [76]. The Sleep Heart Health Study has also reported evidence of vascular dysfunction among older participants, particularly arterial diameter [77]. These investigators have identified OSA as an independent risk factor for impaired flow-mediated vasodilation. However, endothelial dysfunction is often seen in patients with hypertension, hyperlipidemia, diabetes, or smoking; these comorbidities may limit the importance of OSA as an independent risk factor for endothelial dysfunction.

Blood coagulation abnormalities

Increased cardiovascular risk in OSA patients may also be linked to abnormalities of coagulation and excessive platelet activation, and this topic has been recently reviewed [78]. Increased circulating levels of activated coagulation factors have been reported by Robinson and colleagues [79] in untreated OSA patients, but CPAP treatment appeared not to modify them. Interestingly, two groups have recently reported an increased D-dimer level in untreated OSA and its correlation with the severity of nocturnal hypoxemia, suggesting that a hypercoagulable state is potentially involved in cardiovascular risk in OSA patients [80,81]. Other investigators have found increased blood viscosity in untreated adult OSA [82]; increased fibrinogen level in both adults [82] and children with sleep disordered breathing [83]; and evidence of platelet activation which decreased after CPAP treatment [84,85]. However, some uncertainties still remain on the independent role of OSA on increased blood coagulability, because of the common coexistence of other cardiovascular risk factors, the lack of correlation between markers such as fibrinogen and severity of sleep disordered breathing in children, and the incomplete normalization of coagulation after CPAP treatment.

Metabolic dysregulation

There is growing evidence of an association of OSA with the metabolic syndrome. Within this syndrome, obesity, a sedentary lifestyle, and genetic propensity cause insulin resistance, impaired glucose tolerance, and hyperinsulinemia, which further lead to hypertension and dyslipidaemia. A number of positive adverse interactions between these risk factors further increase the cardiovascular risk. OSA-related factors that may contribute to metabolic dysregulation include increased sympathetic activity, sleep fragmentation, and intermittent hypoxia.

Glucose intolerance

The mechanisms of impaired glucose tolerance in OSA particularly involve insulin resistance. A number of reports found increased insulin resistance, impaired glucose tolerance, and dyslipidaemia in OSA patients independent of body weight [86–88], and a worsening of insulin resistance with increasing apnea hypopnea index (AHI) [89]. However, data evaluating the improvement of the metabolic syndrome with CPAP therapy are inconsistent [90–93]. While the primary outcome varied across studies, the general study design was a pre- and post-CPAP evaluation. Most studies were lacking a control group and objective measurements of compliance. Furthermore, the impact of CPAP therapy on insulin sensitivity is unclear, with many reports showing no improvement. One report studied 40 subjects before, after 2 days, and after 3 months of treatment, and demonstrated an improvement in insulin sensitivity in OSA subjects versus controls, but the improvement was mainly noticed in less obese patients (body mass index less than 30 kg/m^2) indicating that obesity is more strongly associated with the development of metabolic disturbances than OSA itself [93].

In nondiabetic OSA patients, circulating advanced glycation end products have been reported to correlate with the severity of intermittent hypoxia [94], and a cause-effect relationship between hypoxia and glucose intolerance has been shown by studies in healthy humans beings [95]. Animal studies also support an important role for intermittent hypoxia in the development of insulin resistance, which appears to be dependent on disruption of leptin pathways [96].

The leptin pathway

OSA may also be associated with abnormalities in metabolism that could predispose to weight gain.

Leptin is an adipocyte-derived hormone that regulates body weight through control of appetite and energy expenditure. Leptin may predispose to platelet aggregation and has been implicated as an independent cardiovascular risk factor [97]. Leptin has also been extensively studied in recent years because of its role in appetite regulation [98], but its functions are probably more complex than initially believed. Human obesity is associated with increased leptin levels and a state of leptin resistance, while lack of leptin causes obesity in animal models [99]. Leptin likely exerts pleiotropic functions in OSA, not only by its effects on metabolism and obesity, but also by affecting ventilatory control [99]. Expression of the human leptin gene is regulated by hypoxia [100]. Hypercapnic OSA patients also show a higher degree of leptin resistance compared with nonhypercapnic subjects [101], and similar data have been reported in obese non-OSA subjects [102].

Several studies have reported that OSA is associated with hyperleptinemia, although some were not adjusted for obesity and visceral fat distribution. One study reported that elevated leptin levels in OSA were only found in obese subjects [103], whereas other studies found that sleep hypoxemia was the principal determinant [104]. A study from the Cleveland family study also demonstrated body mass index to be an important confounding factor in the relationship between OSA and leptin levels [105]. Effective treatment with CPAP has been reported to be associated with a decrease in leptin levels [106,107], although in one study the fall in leptin levels was only observed in nonobese patients [107]. The study of Shimizu and colleagues [108] is particularly interesting in that these investigators related changes in plasma leptin levels to cardiac sympathetic function and, thus, sought to link different pathogenetic mechanisms of cardiovascular complications in OSA. While the results were not conclusive, the findings indicated a significant fall in leptin levels with CPAP therapy. However, another study found that leptin levels, when adjusted for body fat distribution, were not related to indices of OSA [109], and a further study indicated that leptin levels were more closely associated with indices of obesity and lipid dysfunction than with indices of OSA [110]. Thus, the possibility of an independent relationship of leptin and other adipocytokines (such as adiponectin and ghrelin) to OSA requires further investigation.

References

[1] Somers V, Javaheri S. Cardiovascular effects of sleep-related breathing disorders. In: Kryger MH, Roth T, Dement WC, editors.

Principles and Practices of Sleep Medicine. 4th edition. Philadelphia: WB Saunders; 2005. p. 1180–91.

[2] Lavie L. Obstructive sleep apnoea syndrome—an oxidative stress disorder. Sleep Med Rev 2003;7:35–51.

[3] Leuenberger U, Jacob E, Sweer L, et al. Surges of muscle sympathetic nerve activity during obstructive apnea are linked to hypoxemia. J Appl Physiol 1995;79:581–8.

[4] Fletcher EC, Miller J, Schaaf JW, et al. Urinary catecholamines before and after tracheostomy in patients with obstructive sleep apnea and hypertension. Sleep 1987;10(1):35–44.

[5] Ziegler MG, Mills PJ, Loredo JS, et al. Effect of continuous positive airway pressure and placebo treatment on sympathetic nervous activity in patients with obstructive sleep apnea. Chest 2001;120(3):887–93.

[6] Smith ML, Niedermaier ON, Hardy SM, et al. Role of hypoxemia in sleep apnea-induced sympathoexcitation. J Auton Nerv Syst 1996; 56:184–90.

[7] Narkiewicz K, van de Borne PJ, Pesek CA, et al. Selective potentiation of peripheral chemoreflex sensitivity in obstructive sleep apnea. Circulation 1999;99:1183–9.

[8] Hedner J, Ejnell H, Sellgren J, et al. Is high and fluctuating muscle nerve sympathetic activity in the sleep apnoea syndrome of pathogenetic importance for the development of hypertension? J Hypertens Suppl 1988;6:S529–31.

[9] Somers VK, Dyken ME, Clary MP, et al. Sympathetic neural mechanisms in obstructive sleep apnea. J Clin Invest 1995;96:1897–904.

[10] Carlson JT, Hedner J, Elam M, et al. Augmented resting sympathetic activity in awake patients with obstructive sleep apnea. Chest 1993;103: 1763–8.

[11] Narkiewicz K, Kato M, Phillips BG, et al. Nocturnal continuous positive airway pressure decreases daytime sympathetic traffic in obstructive sleep apnea. Circulation 1999;100: 2332–5.

[12] Parati G, Di Rienzo M, Bertinieri G, et al. Evaluation of the baroreceptor-heart rate reflex by 24-hour intra-arterial blood pressure monitoring in humans. Hypertension 1988;12: 214–22.

[13] Bertinieri G, Di Rienzo M, Cavallazzi A, et al. Evaluation of baroreceptors reflex by blood pressure monitoring in unanesthetized cats. Am J Physiol 1988;254:H377–83.

[14] Parati G, Di Rienzo M, Bonsignore MR, et al. Autonomic cardiac regulation in obstructive sleep apnea syndrome: evidence from spontaneous baroreflex analysis during sleep. J Hypertens 1997;15:1621–6.

[15] Bonsignore MR, Parati G, Insalaco G, et al. CPAP treatment improves baroreflex control of heart rate during sleep in severe OSA. Am J Respir Crit Care Med 2002;166:279–86.

[16] Bonsignore MR, Parati G, Insalaco G, et al. Baroreflex control of heart rate during sleep in severe obstructive sleep apnoea: effects of acute CPAP. Eur Respir J 2006;27:128–35.

[17] Ryan S, Ward S, Heneghan C, et al. Predictors of decreased spontaneous baroreflex sensitivity in obstructive sleep apnea syndrome. Chest 2007;131(4):1100–7.

[18] Brooks D, Horner RL, Kozar LF, et al. Obstructive sleep apnea as a cause of systemic hypertension. Evidence from a canine model. J Clin Invest 1997;99:106–9.

[19] Fletcher EC. Physiological consequences of intermittent hypoxia: systemic blood pressure. [invited review]. J Appl Physiol 2001;90:1600–5.

[20] Fletcher EC, Bao G, Li R. Renin activity and blood pressure in response to chronic episodic hypoxia. Hypertension 1999;34:309–14.

[21] Bao G, Metreveli N, Li R, et al. Blood pressure response to chronic episodic hypoxia: role of the sympathetic nervous system. J Appl Physiol 1997;83:95–101.

[22] Willerson JT, Ridker PM. Inflammation as a cardiovascular risk factor. Circulation 2004; 109(21 Suppl 1):II2–10.

[23] Glass CK, Witztum JL. Atherosclerosis: the road ahead. Cell 2001;104(4):503–16.

[24] Blake GJ, Ridker PM. Inflammatory bio-markers and cardiovascular risk prediction. J Intern Med 2002;252(4):283–94.

[25] Kritchevsky SB, Cesari M, Pahor M. Inflammatory markers and cardiovascular health in older adults. Cardiovasc Res 2005;66(2):265–75.

[26] Ghosh S, May MJ, Kopp EB. NF-kappa B and Rel proteins: evolutionarily conserved mediators of immune responses. Annu Rev Immunol 1998;16:225–60.

[27] Skoog T, Dichtl W, Boquist S, et al. Plasma tumour necrosis factor-alpha and early carotid atherosclerosis in healthy middle-aged men. Eur Heart J 2002;23(5):376–83.

[28] Cesari M, Penninx BW, Newman AB, et al. Inflammatory markers and onset of cardiovascular events: results from the Health ABC study. Circulation 2003;108(19):2317–22.

[29] Ridker PM, Rifai N, Pfeffer M, et al. Elevation of tumor necrosis factor-alpha and increased risk of recurrent coronary events after myocardial infarction. Circulation 2000;101(18): 2149–53.

[30] Ciftci TU, Kokturk O, Bukan N, et al. The relationship between serum cytokine levels with obesity and obstructive sleep apnea syndrome. Cytokine 2004;28(2):87–91.

[31] Dyugovskaya L, Lavie P, Lavie L. Phenotypic and functional characterization of blood gamma-delta T cells in sleep apnea. Am J Respir Crit Care Med 2003;168(2):242–9.

[32] Minoguchi K, Tazaki T, Yokoe T, et al. Elevated production of tumor necrosis factor-alpha by monocytes in patients with obstructive sleep apnea syndrome. Chest 2004;126(5):1473–9.

[33] Ryan S, Taylor CT, McNicholas WT. Predictors of elevated nuclear factor-kappaB-dependent genes in obstructive sleep apnea syndrome. Am J Respir Crit Care Med 2006;174(7):824-30.

[34] Riha RL, Brander P, Vennelle M, et al. Tumour necrosis factor-alpha (-308) gene polymorphism in obstructive sleep apnoea-hypopnoea syndrome. Eur Respir J 2005;26(4):673-8.

[35] Ohga E, Tomita T, Wada H, et al. Increased levels of circulating ICAM-1, VCAM-1, and L-selectin in obstructive sleep apnea syndrome. J Appl Physiol 1999;87:10-4.

[36] Blake GJ, Ridker PM. C-reactive protein and other inflammatory risk markers in acute coronary syndromes. J Am Coll Cardiol 2003;41:37-42.

[37] Ridker PM, Hennekens CH, Buring JE, et al. C-reactive protein and other markers of inflammation in the prediction of cardiovascular disease in women. N Engl J Med 2000;342:836-43.

[38] Ridker PM, Cushman M, Stampfer MJ, et al. Plasma concentration of C-reactive protein and risk of developing peripheral vascular disease. Circulation 1998;97:425-8.

[39] Shamsuzzaman AS, Winnicki M, Lanfranchi P, et al. Elevated C-reactive protein in patients with obstructive sleep apnea. Circulation 2002;105:2462-4.

[40] Yokoe T, Minoguchi K, Matsuo H, et al. Elevated levels of C-reactive protein and interleukin-6 in patients with obstructive sleep apnea syndrome are decreased by nasal continuous positive airway pressure. Circulation 2003;107:1129-34.

[41] Tauman R, Ivanenko A, O'Brien LM, et al. Plasma C-reactive protein levels among children with sleep-disordered breathing. Pediatrics 2004;113:564-9.

[42] Punjabi NM, Beamer BA. C-reactive protein is associated with sleep disordered breathing independent of adiposity. Sleep 2007;30(1):29-34.

[43] Guilleminault C, Kirisoglu C, Ohayon MM. C-reactive protein and sleep-disordered breathing. Sleep 2004;27:1507-11.

[44] Athanasios G, Kaditis AG, Alexopoulos EI, et al. Morning levels of C-reactive protein in children with obstructive sleep-disordered breathing. Am J Respir Crit Care Med 2005;171:282-6.

[45] Ryan S, Nolan G, Hannigan E, et al. Cardiovascular risk markers in obstructive sleep apnoea syndrome and correlation with obesity. Thorax 2007;62(6):509-14

[46] Ryan S, Taylor CT, McNicholas WT. Selective activation of inflammatory pathways by intermittent hypoxia in obstructive sleep apnea syndrome. Circulation 2005;112(17):2660-7.

[47] Goldbart A, Row BW, Kheirandish L, et al. Intermittent hypoxic exposure during light phase induces changes in cAMP response element binding protein activity in the rat CA1 hippocampal region: water maze performance correlates. Neuroscience 2003;122:585-90.

[48] Lavie L, Kraiczi H, Hefetz A, et al. Plasma vascular endothelial growth factor in sleep apnea syndrome: effects of nasal continuous positive air pressure treatment. Am J Respir Crit Care Med 2002;165:1624-8.

[49] Schulz R, Mahmoudi S, Hattar K, et al. Enhanced release of superoxide from polymorphonuclear neutrophils in obstructive sleep apnea. Am J Respir Crit Care Med 2000;162:566-70.

[50] Dyugovskaya L, Lavie P, Lavie L. Increased adhesion molecules expression and production of reactive oxygen species in leukocytes of sleep apnea patients. Am J Respir Crit Care Med 2002;165(7):934-9.

[51] Chen L, Einbinder E, Zhang Q, et al. Oxidative stress and left ventricular function with chronic intermittent hypoxia in rats. Am J Respir Crit Care Med 2005;172:915-20.

[52] Xu W, Chi L, Row BW, et al. Increased oxidative stress is associated with chronic intermittent hypoxia-mediated brain cortical neuronal cell apoptosis in a mouse model of sleep apnea. Neuroscience 2004;126:313-23.

[53] Veasey SC, Davis CW, Fenik P, et al. Long-term intermittent hypoxia in mice: protracted hypersomnolence with oxidative injury to sleep-wake brain regions. Sleep 2004;27:194-201.

[54] Zhan G, Serrano F, Fenik P, et al. NADPH oxidase mediates hypersomnolence and brain oxidative injury in a murine model of sleep apnea. Am J Respir Crit Care Med 2005;172:921-9.

[55] Lavie L, Vishnevsky A, Lavie P. Evidence for lipid peroxidation in obstructive sleep apnea. Sleep 2004;27:123-8.

[56] Carpagnano GE, Kharitonov SA, Resta O, et al. 8-Isoprostane, a marker of oxidative stress, is increased in exhaled breath condensate of patients with obstructive sleep apnea after night and is reduced by continuous positive airway pressure therapy. Chest 2003;124:1386-92.

[57] Schulz R, Seeger W, Grimminger F. Serum nitrite/nitrate levels in obstructive sleep apnea. Am J Respir Crit Care Med 2001;164:1997-8.

[58] Zhan G, Fenik P, Pratico D, et al. Inducible nitric oxide synthase in long-term intermittent hypoxia: hypersomnolence and brain injury. Am J Respir Crit Care Med 2005;171:1414-20.

[59] Ross R. Atherosclerosis—an inflammatory disease. N Engl J Med 1999;340:115-26.

[60] Vogel RA. Heads and hearts: the endothelial connection. Circulation 2003;107:2766-8.

[61] Drager LF, Bortolotto LA, Lorenzi MC, et al. Early signs of atherosclerosis in obstructive sleep apnea. Am J Respir Crit Care Med 2005;172:613-8.

[62] Kraiczi H, Hedner J, Peker Y, et al. Increased vasoconstrictor sensitivity in obstructive sleep apnea. J Appl Physiol 2000;89:493-8.

[63] Kato M, Roberts-Thomson P, Phillips BG, et al. Impairment of endothelium-dependent vasodilation of resistance vessels in patients with obstructive sleep apnea. Circulation 2000;102:2607–10.

[64] Ip MS, Tse HF, Lam B, et al. Endothelial function in obstructive sleep apnea and response to treatment. Am J Respir Crit Care Med 2004;169:348–53.

[65] Carlson JT, Rangemark C, Hedner JA. Attenuated endothelium-dependent vascular relaxation in patients with sleep apnoea. J Hypertens 1996;14:77–84.

[66] Duchna HW, Guilleminault C, Stoohs RA, et al. Vascular reactivity in obstructive sleep apnea syndrome. Am J Respir Crit Care Med 2000;161:187–91.

[67] Ohike Y, Kozaki K, Iijima K, et al. Amelioration of vascular endothelial dysfunction in obstructive sleep apnea syndrome by nasal continuous positive airway pressure—possible involvement of nitric oxide and asymmetric NG, NG-dimethylarginine. Circ J 2005;69:221–6.

[68] Faulx MD, Larkin EK, Hoit BD, et al. Sex influences endothelial function in sleep-disordered breathing. Sleep 2004;27:1113–20.

[69] Joyner MJ, Dietz NM. Nitric oxide and vasodilation in human limbs. J Appl Physiol 1997;83:1785–96.

[70] Schulz R, Schmidt D, Blum A, et al. Decreased plasma levels of nitric oxide derivatives in obstructive sleep apnoea: response to CPAP therapy. Thorax 2000;55:1046–51.

[71] Ip MS, Lam B, Chan LY, et al. Circulating nitric oxide is suppressed in obstructive sleep apnea and is reversed by nasal continuous positive airway pressure. Am J Respir Crit Care Med 2000;162:2166–71.

[72] Agusti AG, Barbe F, Togores B. Exhaled nitric oxide in patients with sleep apnea. Sleep 1999;22:231–5.

[73] Haight JS, Djupesland PG. Nitric oxide (NO) and obstructive sleep apnea (OSA). Sleep Breath 2003;7:53–62.

[74] Olopade CO, Zakkar M, Swedler WI, et al. Exhaled pentane and nitric oxide levels in patients with obstructive sleep apnea. Chest 1997;111:1500–4.

[75] Phillips BG, Narkiewicz K, Pesek CA, et al. Effects of obstructive sleep apnea on endothelin-1 and blood pressure. J Hypertens 1999;17:61–6.

[76] Grimpen F, Kanne P, Schulz E, et al. Endothelin-1 plasma levels are not elevated in patients with obstructive sleep apnoea. Eur Respir J 2000;15:320–5.

[77] Nieto FJ, Herrington DM, Redline S, et al. Sleep apnea and markers of vascular endothelial function in a large community sample of older adults. Am J Respir Crit Care Med 2004;169:354–60.

[78] von Kanel R, Dimsdale JE. Hemostatic alterations in patients with obstructive sleep apnea and the implications for cardiovascular disease. Chest 2003;124:1956–67.

[79] Robinson GV, Pepperell JC, Segal HC, et al. Circulating cardiovascular risk factors in obstructive sleep apnoea: data from randomised controlled trials. Thorax 2004;59:777–82.

[80] Shitrit D, Peled N, Shitrit AB, et al. An association between oxygen desaturation and D-dimer in patients with obstructive sleep apnea syndrome. Thromb Haemost 2005;94:544–7.

[81] Von Kanel R, Loredo JS, Powell FL, et al. Short-term isocapnic hypoxia and coagulation activation in patients with sleep apnea. Clin Hemorheol Microcirc 2005;33:369–77.

[82] Steiner S, Jax T, Evers S, et al. Altered blood rheology in obstructive sleep apnea as a mediator of cardiovascular risk. Cardiology 2005;104:92–6.

[83] Kaditis AG, Alexopoulos EI, Kalampouka E, et al. Morning levels of fibrinogen in children with sleep-disordered breathing. Eur Respir J 2004;24:790–7.

[84] Shimizu M, Kamio K, Haida M, et al. Platelet activation in patients with obstructive sleep apnea syndrome and effects of nasal-continuous positive airway pressure. Tokai J Exp Clin Med 2002;27:107–12.

[85] Hui DS, Ko FW, Fok JP, et al. The effects of nasal continuous positive airway pressure on platelet activation in obstructive sleep apnea syndrome. Chest 2004;125:1768–75.

[86] Strohl KP, Novak RD, Singer W, et al. Insulin levels, blood pressure and sleep apnea. Sleep 1994;17(7):614–8.

[87] Ip MS, Lam B, Ng MM, et al. Obstructive sleep apnea is independently associated with insulin resistance. Am J Respir Crit Care Med 2002;165(5):670–6.

[88] Vgontzas AN, Papanicolaou DA, Bixler EO, et al. Sleep apnea and daytime sleepiness and fatigue: relation to visceral obesity, insulin resistance, and hypercytokinemia. J Clin Endocrinol Metab 2000;85(3):1151–8.

[89] Punjabi NM, Sorkin JD, Katzel LI, et al. Sleep-disordered breathing and insulin resistance in middle-aged and overweight men. Am J Respir Crit Care Med 2002;165(5):677–82.

[90] Brooks B, Cistulli PA, Borkman M, et al. Obstructive sleep apnea in obese noninsulin-dependent diabetic patients: effect of continuous positive airway pressure treatment on insulin responsiveness. J Clin Endocrinol Metab 1994;79(6):1681–5.

[91] Saarelainen S, Lahtela J, Kallonen E. Effect of nasal CPAP treatment on insulin sensitivity and plasma leptin. J Sleep Res 1997;6(2):146–7.

[92] Smurra M, Philip P, Taillard J, et al. CPAP treatment does not affect glucose-insulin metabolism in sleep apneic patients. Sleep Med 2001;2(3):207–13.

[93] Harsch IA, Schahin SP, Radespiel-Troger M, et al. Continuous positive airway pressure

treatment rapidly improves insulin sensitivity in patients with obstructive sleep apnea syndrome. Am J Respir Crit Care Med 2004; 169(2):156–62.

[94] Tan KC, Chow WS, Lam JC, et al. Advanced glycation endproducts in nondiabetic patients with obstructive sleep apnea. Sleep 2006;29: 329–33.

[95] Oltmanns KM, Gehring H, Rudolf S, et al. Hypoxia causes glucose intolerance in humans. Am J Respir Crit Care Med 2004;169:1231–7.

[96] Polotsky VY, Li J, Punjabi NM, et al. Intermittent hypoxia increases insulin resistance in genetically obese mice. J Physiol 2003;552: 253–64.

[97] Soderberg S, Ahren B, Jansson JH, et al. Leptin is associated with increased risk of myocardial infarction. J Intern Med 1999;246:409–18.

[98] Greenberg AS, Obin MS. Obesity and the role of adipose tissue in inflammation and metabolism [review]. Am J Clin Nutr 2006;83: 461S–5S.

[99] O'Donnell CP, Tankersley CG, Polotsky VP, et al. Leptin, obesity, and respiratory function [review]. Respir Physiol 2000;119:163–70.

[100] Ambrosini G, Nath AK, Sierra-Honigmann MR, et al. Transcriptional activation of the human leptin gene in response to hypoxia. J Biol Chem 2002;77:34601–9.

[101] Shimura R, Tatsumi K, Nakamura A, et al. Fat accumulation, leptin, and hypercapnia in obstructive sleep apnea-hypopnea syndrome. Chest 2005;127:543–9.

[102] Phipps PR, Starritt E, Caterson I, et al. Association of serum leptin with hypoventilation in human obesity. Thorax 2002;57:75–6.

[103] Barcelo A, Barbe F, Llompart E, et al. Neuropeptide Y and leptin in patients with obstructive sleep apnea syndrome: role of obesity. Am J Respir Crit Care Med 2005;171:183–7.

[104] Tatsumi K, Kasahara Y, Kurosu K, et al. Sleep oxygen desaturation and circulating leptin in obstructive sleep apnea-hypopnea syndrome. Chest 2005;127:716–21.

[105] Patel SR, Palmer LJ, Larkin EK, et al. Relationship between obstructive sleep apnea and diurnal leptin rhythms. Sleep 2004;27:235–9.

[106] Sanner BM, Kollhosser P, Buechner N, et al. Influence of treatment on leptin levels in patients with obstructive sleep apnoea. Eur Respir J 2004;23:601–4.

[107] Harsch IA, Konturek PC, Koebnick C, et al. Leptin and ghrelin levels in patients with obstructive sleep apnoea: effect of CPAP treatment. Eur Respir J 2003;22:251–7.

[108] Shimizu K, Chin K, Nakamura T, et al. Plasma leptin levels and cardiac sympathetic function in patients with obstructive sleep apnoea-hypopnoea syndrome. Thorax 2002;57:429–34.

[109] Schafer H, Pauleit D, Sudhop T, et al. Body fat distribution, serum leptin, and cardiovascular risk factors in men with obstructive sleep apnea. Chest 2002;122:829–39.

[110] Ip MS, Lam KS, Ho C, et al. Serum leptin and vascular risk factors in obstructive sleep apnea. Chest 2000;118:580–6.

SLEEP
MEDICINE
CLINICS

Sleep Med Clin 2 (2007) 549–557

Systemic and Pulmonary Arterial Hypertension in Obstructive Sleep Apnea

Heinrich F. Becker, MD[a,b],*, Shahrokh Javaheri, MD[c]

- Systemic arterial hypertension
  Epidemiology
  Physiologic effects of sleep on blood
    pressure
  Effects of OSA on nighttime blood
    pressure
  Effects of OSA on daytime blood pressure
  Endothelial dysfuction

- Treatment effects
  How might these discrepant results be
    explained?
- Pulmonary arterial hypertension
  Epidemiology
  Is PAH caused by OSA reversible?
- References

Systemic arterial hypertension

Epidemiology

In the early days of research into obstructive sleep apnea (OSA), it became clear that cardiovascular disturbances were highly prevalent among patients with sleep disordered breathing, the most prevalent cardiovascular disorder being arterial hypertension [1]. However, the question of whether OSA is an independent risk factor for arterial hypertension, or if the increased prevalence of hypertension in OSA patients is simply a result of the high prevalence of obesity, physical inactivity, diabetes, smoking, and other factors, was discussed for many years. Based on biologic plausibility, animal experiments, and human studies accounting for confounding factors. There is now clear evidence that OSA is an important and an independent risk factor for hypertension [2].

Several excellent articles from the Wisconsin Sleep Cohort Study of middle-aged state employees demonstrated the fact that OSA is an independent risk factor for arterial hypertension. Young and colleagues [3], accounting for all known confounders, found an increased prevalence of hypertension with increasing OSA severity as measured by the apnea-hypopnea index (AHI, number of events per hour of sleep). In a longitudinal survey of the study participants, Peppard and colleagues [4] demonstrated that the incidence of newly diagnosed arterial hypertension in a 4 year follow-up period increased with the AHI at baseline: in the four groups (AHI of 0, 0.1–4.9, 5–14.9, and 15 or more) there was a 4-year incidence of newly diagnosed hypertension of 9.7%, 17.1%, 31.5%, and 32.1%, respectively [4]. After the adjustment of known risk factors for hypertension, there was still

[a] Philipps-University Marburg
[b] Division of Pulmonary and Critical Care Medicine, AK Barmbek, 22291 Hamburg, Germany
[c] Sleepcare Diagnostics, 4780 Socialville-Fosters Road, Mason, OH 45040, USA
* Corresponding author. Division of Pulmonary and Critical Care Medicine, AK Barmbek, 22291 Hamburg, Germany.
E-mail address: he.becker@asklepios.com (H.F. Becker).

1556-407X/07/$ – see front matter © 2007 Elsevier Inc. All rights reserved.
sleep.theclinics.com

doi:10.1016/j.jsmc.2007.07.010

a two-fold risk increase for subjects with an AHI of 5 to 15 per hour, and a three-fold increase in subjects with an AHI greater than 15, as compared with subjects without breathing disorders at baseline. Several other studies also demonstrated an increased risk of hypertension in patients with OSA independent of other confounding factors, although the risk increase attributed to OSA varied [5–7].

From a clinical point of view it is important to note that even mild OSA, in the AHI range of 5 to 15 per hour, will increase the risk for hypertension. The question as to whether there is a further risk increase in more severe disease with AHI values of 30 or more cannot be answered in the epidemiologic studies mentioned, as these studies are underpowered because of the small number of severely affected subjects. A small further increase in blood pressure was demonstrated in a prospectively studied patient group from a sleep clinic including more than 2,600 subjects [8]. After adjustment for confounders, there was an increase in systolic and diastolic blood pressure of 1 mm Hg and 0.7 mm Hg, respectively, with every AHI increase of 10 per hour. In another large study of 1,087 sleep clinic subjects, there was a similar incidence of high blood pressure in AHI groups of 5 to 20, 20 to 40, and more than 40 subjects. However, the odds ratio of badly controlled hypertension (greater or equal to 160/95 mm Hg) was 4.15 in subjects with an AHI of more than 40, and only 1.5 to 2.15 in subjects with mild or moderate disease, as compared with subjects without sleep apnea [9].

Another interesting finding is that the influence of OSA is more pronounced in nonobese, as compared with obese, subjects [3]. However, this finding might be explained by the statistical over adjustment for the confounder obesity.

The effect of age and gender

In two studies there was a sufficient number of older subjects [5,7]. Both studies demonstrated a risk reduction for the development of hypertension in older subjects, and no risk increase at the age of 65 [7] or 70 [5] and older, respectively. As OSA is an important factor that increases mortality, especially in young patients [10], the lack of an association of OSA and hypertension might simply reflect a strong survival bias of those OSA patients that are less susceptible to hypertension.

Except for the sleep heart health study [5] all other studies did not find an influence of gender on blood pressure risk caused by OSA [3,4,7].

Physiologic effects of sleep on blood pressure

In healthy subjects, the transition from wakefulness to non-rapid eye movement sleep (NREM) is characterized by an increase in parasympathetic drive and a reduction in sympathetic activity. As a consequence, heart rate, arterial blood pressure, cardiac output, and stroke volume decrease, resulting in an overall cardiac workload is reduced, as compared with a subject lying supine during wakefulness [11–13], as blood pressure and cardiac output decrease during sleep. During rapid eye movement (REM) sleep, electroencephalographic (EEG) patterns resemble that of wakefulness, but there is marked muscle atonia and intermittent REM. Not only the EEG pattern is similar to quiet wakefulness, but heart rate, blood pressure, and sympathetic activity also increase to levels that are present during relaxed wakefulness [11,12,14].

Effects of OSA on nighttime blood pressure

Obstructive sleep apnea is characterized by repetitive apneas caused by upper airway collapse during sleep, despite respiratory efforts of the diaphragm. Five or more apneas per hour of sleep are generally considered abnormal, and severely affected patients have several hundred apneas each night, leading to repetitive hypoxia and hypercapnia. The acute consequences of the apneas are hypoxia and hypercapnia, as well as negative intrathoracic pressure during obstructed breaths. Most apneas and hypopneas are terminated by a transient arousal from sleep and consecutive hyperventilation. Disruption of normal sleep by frequent arousals leads to excessive daytime sleepiness, the most prominent symptom in these patients. Both arousals and blood gas changes lead to acute sympathetic activation [11,14] and an increase in heart rate and blood pressure (Fig. 1) that is most prominent during the postapneic hyperventilation. Sympathetic activity during sleep—measured both directly at the peroneal muscle (sympathetic muscle nerve activity) or as norepinephrine in blood or urine—is markedly increased in OSA patients [14–17].

Unlike what one might expect, even in severe OSA the physiologic blood pressure drop during sleep is preserved in most patients. However, mean blood pressure values are significantly higher in an OSA group, compared with subjects without OSA [7].

Effects of OSA on daytime blood pressure

Daytime arterial hypertension is present in up to 60% of OSA patients. The question by which mechanism the acute blood pressure changes during sleep leads to daytime hypertension is still not completely understood. Repetitive episodes of hypoxia are certainly very important in the pathogenesis of daytime hypertension, as they cause sympathetic activation that persists much longer than the actual hypoxic challenge [18,19] and that can be

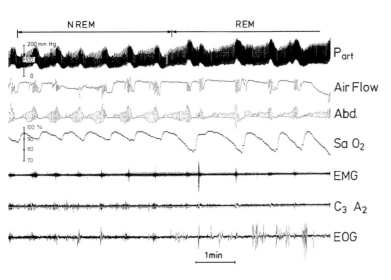

Fig. 1. Invasive blood pressure recording during polysomnography in a patient with severe OSA. Typical mixed apneas of up to 1-minute duration with marked desaturations are present. Toward the end of the apneas there is an increase in arterial blood pressure and a further marked increase after the resumption of breathing. Both blood pressure increase and desaturations are more pronounced during REM-sleep as compared with NREM-sleep. Abd, abdominal movements; Air flow, oro-nasal air flow; C3–A2, Electroencephalogram; ECG, Electrocardiogram; EMG, Electromyogram; Part, arterial blood pressure; SaO₂, arterial oxygen saturation.

prevented by the administration of supplemental oxygen [20]. In an animal model, it has been shown that both acoustic arousal and apnea-induced arousal acutely increase blood pressure to a similar extent. However, only in animals with apneas and consecutive hypoxia was there an increase in daytime blood pressure [21]. Therefore, most likely the most important mechanism causing daytime hypertension is sympathetic activation caused by repetitive hypoxemia, and probably also hypercapnia. Repetitive arousals will increase blood pressure acutely, but a long-term blood pressure increase during daytime does not seem to occur. Apnea related negative intrathoracic pressure swings and hypoxic pulmonary vasoconstriction lead to an increased right heart load. As a consequence, nocturnal atrial natriuretic peptide (ANP) levels are increased and, because of the relative hypervolemia, renin levels are suppressed in OSA patients [22,23]. These changes might contribute to the pathogenesis of daytime hypertension. With nasal continuous positive airway pressure (CPAP) therapy, renin levels increase and ANP levels decrease during sleep [22,23].

Endothelial dysfunction

In patients with sleep apnea, endothelial dysfunction may be the link between increased sympathetic activity, hypoxia and elevated blood pressure. Nitric oxide (NO), the most potent biologic vasodilator, is decreased and asymmetric dimethyl arginin levels, the physiologic NO antagonist, as well as endothelin, the most potent vasoconstrictor, are elevated [24,25]. Vascular reactivity is attenuated in OSA patients: the infusion of isoprenalin, an alpha- and

β-mimetic drug, or angiotensin II cause a smaller blood flow change in OSA patients as compared with normal subjects [26,27]. A variety of biochemical changes, as markers of endothelial dysfunction, have been shown in OSA patients, as compared with normal subjects, and the reversibility of these changes with effective treatment has also been demonstrated [24,28,29]. Reduced vascular reactivity and endothelial dysfunction, as a consequence of chronic sympathetic activation and repetitive hypoxia and reoxygenation, might be the link between sleep apnea and daytime hypertension and atherosclerosis in the long term.

Treatment effects

With the proven strong association of arterial hypertension and OSA, one would expect a substantial blood pressure reduction with effective treatment of OSA. In fact, numerous uncontrolled studies in the pre "evidence based medicine era" have shown a marked blood pressure reduction—both during nighttime and daytime—with CPAP treatment in OSA patients. However, controlled studies have demonstrated conflicting results. There was no significant drop in mean arterial blood pressure with CPAP treatment in five studies [30–34], and a small decrease in diastolic (−1.4 mm Hg) [35] or diastolic and mean daytime blood pressure, by approximately 2 mm Hg [36]. Only three studies demonstrated a relevant reduction of mean blood pressure by 2.5 mm Hg [37], approximately 6 mm Hg [38], and 9.9 mm Hg on average, respectively [39]. The drop in mean 24-hour blood pressure was not only because of a reduction of nighttime blood pressure, but to a similar extent also because of a decrease of daytime blood pressure (Fig. 2).

How might these discrepant results be explained?

Percentage of hypertensive patients in the different studies

The most important difference in the studies published so far is the number of hypertensive patients included. In a normotensive OSA patient a marked blood pressure (BP) decrease during daytime cannot be expected. In four of the six studies that showed no or only little effect on mean BP [30,32,33,35], the percentage of hypertensive subjects was 0%, 25%, 25%, and 38% respectively, whereas the number of hypertensive subjects has not been reported in the other two articles [31,34]. The prevalence of arterial hypertension was only slightly higher than that in the general population. In the study that showed the largest effect [39], 66% of subjects were hypertensive. The subgroup analysis by Pepperell and colleagues [37], examining the 22 patients that were on antihypertensive medication (11 patients each in the CPAP and sham group, with similar baseline AHI) showed a substantial reduction in blood pressure (−7.9 mm Hg) in those patients treated with CPAP, and only a mild decrease (−1.2 mm Hg) in the sham group.

In a group of 11 OSA patients with refractory hypertension, treatment with CPAP for 2 months (in an uncontrolled design) lowered 24-hour systolic and diastolic BP by 11 mm Hg and 7.8 mm Hg, respectively [40]. Heitmann and colleagues compared the effect of CPAP in ten normotensive and eight hypertensive OSA patients, using invasive blood pressure recording (uncontrolled design) and found a mild reduction in 24-hour BP by 1.9 mm Hg in normotensives and a 8 mm Hg decrease in the

hypertensives with optimal treatment for 6 weeks [17]. In summary, all these data suggest that there is a small effect of nasal CPAP in normotensive OSA patients, especially during nighttime. In contrast, a clinically important reduction in BP can be demonstrated in hypertensive patients.

Severity of OSA

The subgroup analysis in two studies demonstrated a reduction in blood pressure in patients with more than 33 desaturations per hour or more than 20 desaturations per hour of at least 4%, compared with patients who did not fulfil these severity criteria [35,37]. In the studies in mild OSA [31,33] there was no effect of treatment on blood pressure. In summary, in more severe sleep apnea the effect of treatment seems to be more pronounced.

Compliance, duration, and effectiveness of treatment

Patients with a CPAP use of less than 5 hours per night did not experience a blood pressure reduction, whereas this was the case in patients with more than 5 hours of use [37]. In one study the treatment period was only 1 week [32], which seems too short, given the fact that most studies of antihypertensives use a treatment period of at least 4 weeks.

With the exception of two studies [37,39], the effects of treatment on AHI have not been reported, and in these two studies there was a substantial decrease in AHI in the "sham" group. Therefore, in the sham group of other studies there may well have been a treatment effect, leading to blood pressure reduction in the control group.

Method of blood pressure recording

Discontinuous ambulatory BP monitoring leads to arousal and will overestimate nighttime blood

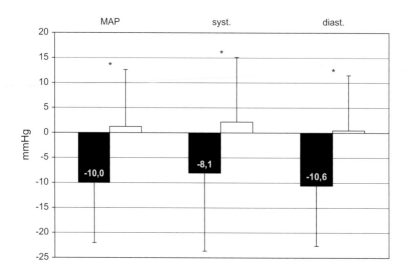

Fig. 2. Daytime blood pressure changes with effective (*closed bars*) and subtherapeutic CPAP.

pressure. Continuous noninvasive recording has a very high correlation with invasively measured blood pressure and is certainly the most accurate noninvasive method. In the study that used continuous recording [39], the blood pressure reduction was most pronounced.

Number of patients treated and statistical power

Most studies did not include a statistical power analysis. It is certainly very difficult if not impossible to calculate statistical power in normotensive patients. Both studies that had a power analysis showed a significant blood pressure reduction with treatment [37,39].

Influence of excessive daytime sleepiness

Two studies in asymptomatic OSA patients with fairly severe OSA did not find an effect of OSA treatment on blood pressure [34,41] studied asymptomatic patients with fairly severe OSA (AHI aproximately 55 per hour and 28 desaturations greater than 4%, respectively). Most of the subjects in the Barbé and colleagues [38] study were normotensive and a blood pressure reduction would not be expected in these subjects. However, the Oxford group [41] studied hypertensive, nonsleepy patients and still they did not find a blood pressure reduction with CPAP. One might therefore come to the conclusion that in patients without symptoms there is no effect of treatment on blood pressure. Most of these nonsleepy OSA patients, however, were on antihypertensive treatment and their hypertension was well controlled.

Sham treatment used?

The sham treatment used does not seem to influence results a great deal. If a mask with a low pressure is used, there may be a treatment effect that would act against the hypothesis of blood pressure reduction, as the sham group would also be at least partly treated [39]. In any case, if low mask pressure is used as a sham treatment, the effect on AHI should be determined upon treatment.

Is there an effect of CPAP on arterial hypertension and what is the effect size?

Most studies did not show an effect of CPAP on blood pressure. However, all of the negative studies had the severe limitations that they were underpowered, as subjects were mainly or exclusively normotensive. In addition, treatment duration was too short or compliance inadequate.

Critical evaluation of the data available at present leads to the conclusion that

1. In hypertensive patients with moderate to severe sleep apnea there is a blood pressure drop by approximately 10 mm Hg on average with CPAP treatement;
2. In less severe OSA, this blood pressure lowering effect will be smaller;
3. Even in normotensive OSA patients, there is a mild reduction in daytime blood pressure by 1 mm Hg to 2 mm Hg; and
4. The effect on blood pressure requires effective treatment and adequate compliance.

Pulmonary arterial hypertension

Epidemiology

In 1998, the second World Health Organization conference on pulmonary arterial hypertension (PAH) [42] recognized sleep disordered breathing as a secondary cause of PAH. In patients with OSA, the prevalence of PAH varies from about 15% to 70% [2,43], and is usually mild at rest, but could be severe enough, resulting in cor pulmonale, a feature of Pickwickian syndrome (hypercapnic OSA syndrome). Pulmonary hypertension gets worse with exercise and may result in dyspnea and exercise intolerance.

Cyclic nocturnal PAH was demonstrated in an early study [44] of 12 subjects with OSA who had undergone right heart catherization. Marked degree of recurrent hypoxemia and hypercapnia was associated with hemodynamic abnormalities. In some of these subjects, systolic pulmonary artery pressure (PAP) exceeded 60 mm Hg. During wakefulness, four subjects had mild PAH, and mean pressure ranged from 20 mm Hg to 22 mm Hg. One of these four subjects had an elevated pulmonary capillary wedge pressure (PCWP) of 16 mm Hg. With exercise, most of the subjects developed PAH with mean pulmonary artery pressure of about 30 mm Hg. In some of these subjects, the wedge pressure increased with exercise, unmasking underlying left ventricular diastolic dysfunction. This study indicated that OSA impaired the physiologic processes that normally operate to enable pulmonary circulation, and left ventricular function to maintain pulmonary artery pressure close to normal in the face of increases in cardiac output.

There are a number of studies [45–48] which demonstrated that PAH is relatively common in patients with OSA (Box 1). The first three studies [45–47] used full night polysomnography and right heart catheterization, the gold standard for diagnosis of OSA and PAH. In a French study [45] involving 220 consecutive subjects with AHI greater than 20, 37 subjects (17%) had resting mean pulmonary artery pressure of at least 20 mm Hg (range 20 mm Hg to 44 mm Hg). Patients with PAH had more severe OSA, a higher $Paco_2$, a higher body mass index, and a lower Pao_2 than patients without PAH.

Box 1: Pulmonary arterial hypertension in obstructive sleep apnea

Chaouat and colleagues [45]

- 220 consecutive patients with AHI greater than 20 per hour
- 17% had mean PAP greater than 20 mm Hg
- Patients with PAH had more severe OSA, higher $Paco_2$ and body mass index (BMI), lower Pao_2, and more obstructive and restrictive defect
- $Paco_2$ and forced expiratory volume in the FEV_1 were independent predictors of PAH

Laks and colleagues [46]

- 100 consecutive patients with AHI greater than 20 per hour
- 42% had mean PAP greater than 20 mm Hg; range, 20 mm Hg to 52 mm Hg
- $Paco_2$, Pao_2, and FEV_1 accounted for 33% of variability in PAH

Sanner and colleagues [47]

- 92 consecutive patients with OSA and AHI greater than 10 per hour; (range, 10–100 per hour)
- Chronic obstructive pulminary disease (COPD) was an exclusion criterion
- 20% had mild PAH; range, 20 mm Hg to 25 mm Hg
- Eight subjects had increased PCWP; all had systemic hypertension
- PCWP and time greater than 90% saturation were independent predictors of PAH

Arias and colleagues [48]

- 23 OSA subjects (AHI equals 44 per hour) without any known comorbid disorders
- 43% of the OSA subjects had pulmonary artery systolic hypertension compared with none in the control group (n = 10)
- Subjects with PASH had severe OSA (AHI equals 69 per hour) compared with OSA subjects without PASH (AHI equals 25 per hour)
- 12 weeks effective treatment with CPAP significantly decreased PASH (pulmonary artery systolic decreased 8.5 mm Hg in OSA subjects with baseline PASH)

Furthermore, patients with PAH had higher prevalence of both obstructive and restrictive pulmonary defects. $Paco_2$ and first second of expiration (FEV_1) were the two major predictors of PAH.

In an Australian study [46] of 100 consecutive subjects with an AHI of 20 or more, 42% had PAH, with the mean pulmonary artery pressure ranging from about 20 mm Hg to 52 mm Hg. In this study $Paco_2$, Pao_2, and FEV_1 accounted for

about 33% of variability in pulmonary artery pressure. Six patients with PAH had normal Pao_2.

In a German study [47] of 92 consecutive subjects with AHI greater than 10, and using COPD as an exclusion criterion, 20% had mild PAH with a mean pulmonary artery pressure of 20 mm Hg to 25 mm Hg. Eight subjects had increased PCWP, and all of these subjects had systemic hypertension that was presumably causing left ventricular diastolic dysfunction. Pulmonary capillary wedge pressure and time spent below saturation of 90% were the independent variables predicting PAH.

Presence of PAH in patients with OSA but without COPD has also been confirmed in a French study [49]. COPD was defined as an FEV_1 of less than 70% predicted and FEV_1/FVC ratio of less than 60% predicted. In this study [49] involving 44 subjects, 12 subjects (27%) had precapillary PAH. The inivestigators reported that mean pulmonary artery pressure was positively correlated with BMI and negatively correlated with Pao_2 [49]. Subjects with PAH had significantly lower values for FVC and FEV_1. The mechanisms by which BMI positively correlated with PAH could have been multifactorial and related to restrictive lung defect and hypoxemia.

In conclusion, mild PAH is common in patients with OSA and may occur in the absence of COPD as well as daytime hypoxemia. However, severe OSA, severe hypoxemia, and obstructive or restrictive lung defects are more commonly associated with PAH.

Mechanisms of PAH in OSA

Multiple mechanisms mediate nocturnal rises in pulmonary artery pressure [2]. These include alterations in blood gases, cardiac output, lung volume, intrathoracic pressure, compliance of pulmonary circulation, and left ventricular diastolic dysfunction. In regard to diural PAH, it could be precapillary or postcapillary in nature (see Box 1). Postcapillary PAH could be caused by left ventricular hypertrophy and diastolic dysfunction caused by diurnal systemic hypertension. However, left ventricular hypertrophy could be present in OSA even in the absence of daytime systemic hypertension [50], presumably because of nocturnal cyclic changes in aortic blood pressure and hypoxemia during sleep [51]. In the presence of hypertrophied stiff left ventricle, end-diastolic pressure increases, resulting in an increase in pulmonary capillary, pulmonary artery systolic, and diastolic pressures (postcapillary PAH). Left ventricular diastolic dysfunction may be particularly unmasked when cardiac output increases during exercise, accounting for high prevalence of PAH during exercise observed in patients with OSA [52], and resulting in exertional dyspnea and exercise intolerance.

Loss of vascular surface area, as may occur in COPD, could be an important cause of capillary PAH in patients with OSA. Several studies [45,46,53] have shown that COPD and a low FEV_1 are predictors of PAH in patients with OSA. COPD could also contribute to PAH by way of hypoxemia and hypercapnia, resulting in precapillary PAH (see below).

Finally, an important mechanism contributing to or mediating PAH in OSA is the presence of factors that cause constriction of pulmonary arterioles, which leads to precapillary PAH. The best-known stimulus is alveolar hypoxia, and hypoxemia is an independent predictor of PAH in OSA. However, hypercapnia and changes in intrathoracic pressure could also increase pulmonary arterial blood pressure.

The mechanisms by which hypoxia causes PAH are probably multifactorial and could be related to an imbalance between concentrations of local vasodilators and vasoconstrictors as occurs in endothelial dysfunction syndrome. Furthermore, it is conceivable that if OSA is longstanding, pulmonary vascular remodeling, similar to that in COPD could occur.

Even though cyclic PAH occurs regularly with episodes of apnea during sleep, it is not clear why only some patients with OSA develop diurnal PAH. The same is true for systemic hypertension. It is conceivable that genetic predisposition and polymorphism could be one contributing factor.

In summary, the consequence of OSA on pulmonary circulation may vary from those of cyclic nocturnal PAH, which occurs in virtually all patients, to daytime PAH, right ventricular dysfunction, and eventually cor pulmonale, a feature of Pickwickian syndrome. However, even in the absence of cor pulmonale, which is the manifestation of longstanding severe PAH, presence of PAH increases right ventricular afterload and myocardial oxygen consumption. If PAH develops as a result of increases in cardiac output, for example with exercise, it may cause dyspnea and exercise intolerance.

Is PAH caused by OSA reversible?

Because mechanisms of PAH in OSA are multifactorial, the behavioral response of pulmonary circulation to treatment of OSA with CPAP depends on several factors. For example, if PAH is in part caused by loss of vascular surface area (capillary PAH) because of the presence of a comorbid pathology (COPD or interstitial lung diseases), this component is irreversible. Similarly, if remodeling of the pulmonary vascular bed has occurred, longstanding effective therapy is necessary for reverse remodeling to occur. Therefore, if CPAP is used to treat OSA, long-term adherence with therapy is critical.

Meanwhile, there are several studies suggesting that effective treatment of OSA improves PAH.

Motta and colleagues [54] studied six subjects with severe OSA before and after tracheostomy. After tracheostomy, the mean pulmonary artery pressure decreased significantly by about 50% from 45 mm Hg to 22 mm Hg.

Alchanatis and colleagues [55] used Doppler echocardiography to estimate pulmonary artery pressure before and after 6 months of effective treatment with CPAP in 29 subjects with OSA and without COPD. In six subjects with mild PAH, the mean pulmonary artery pressure decreased significantly, from about 26 mm Hg to 20 mm Hg, 6 months after treatment with CPAP.

Sajkov and colleagues [56], using Doppler echocardiography, studied pulmonary hemodynamics in 20 subjects with OSA (average AHI equals 49) who had normal lung function tests. In this study, CPAP compliance was objectively monitored and the average was 5 hours per night. Patients had normal lung function. Five patients who had mild PAH (range 20 mm Hg to 32 mm Hg) showed the most dramatic decrease in the pulmonary artery pressure, all decreasing below 20 mm Hg after 4 months of effective treatment with CPAP. In a subject who was not compliant with CPAP, there was no change in pulmonary artery pressure. Although this was a single observation, this finding and those reported for systemic hypertension strongly indicate that effective use of CPAP is necessary to lower systemic and pulmonary artery pressures.

So far, the most systematic study has been reported by Arias and colleagues (see Box 1) [48]. This was a randomized clinical trial with sham CPAP. The study involved 23 subjects with severe OSA (AHI equals 44 per hour) and free from any known comorbid disorders. Effective CPAP therapy (6.2 hours per night) for 12 weeks, resulted in a significant decrease in pulmonary artery systolic blood pressure (PASP) from 29 mm Hg to 24 mm Hg (the whole group). The number of patients with PAH decreased from 38% to 14% with CPAP treatment. For these who had PAH at baseline, treatment with CPAP resulted in a clinically and statistically significant drop in PASP (-8.5 mm Hg). In those without baseline PASH, pressure decreased -2.8 mm Hg. Presence of left ventricular diastolic dysfunction also predicted a meaningful drop in pulmonary artery pressure (-7 mm Hg).

The authors should also note that negative studies have been reported. In the study by Sforza and colleagues [57], there were eight subjects with mean PAP equal to 23 mm Hg. After treatment with CPAP for a year, the mean pulmonary artery pressure was 21 mm Hg. For such a small change to be statistically significant, a large sample of patients is necessary. Furthermore, as is the case with systemic hypertension, the authors speculate that with treatment of OSA, a clinically significant drop in pulmonary artery pressure occurs primarily in those patients with higher OSA-related PAH [48].

In summary, the authors conclude that like systemic arterial hypertension, treatment of OSA with CPAP improves pulmonary artery hypertnsion. The drop in blood pressure is particularly more apt to occur in: (1) those with severe OSA, (2) those in whom hypertension (both pulmonary and systemic) is caused by OSA and not caused by a comorbid disorder, (3) those in whom CPAP has been shown to have eliminated OSA, and (4) those who are adherent to CPAP.

References

[1] Coccagna G, Mantovani M, Brignani F, et al. Continuous recording of the pulmonary arterial pressure during sleep in syndromes of hypersomnia with periodic breathing. Bull Physiopathol Respir (Nancy) 1972;8(5):1159–72.

[2] Young T, Javaheri S. Systemic and pulmonary hypertension in obstructive sleep apnea. In: Kryger MH, Roth T, Dement WC, editors. Principles and practices of sleep medicine. 4th edition. Philadelphia: WB Saunders; 2005. p. 1192–202.

[3] Young T, Peppard P, Palta M, et al. Population-based study of sleep-disordered breathing as a risk factor for hypertension. Arch Intern Med 1997;157:1746–52.

[4] Peppard PE, Young T, Palta M, et al. Prospective study of the association between sleep-disordered breathing and hypertension. N Engl J Med 2000;342(19):1378–84.

[5] Bixler EO, Vgontzas AN, Lin HM, et al. Association of hypertension and sleep-disordered breathing. Arch Intern Med 2000;160(15):2289–95.

[6] Duran J, Esnaola S, Rubio R, et al. Obstructive sleep apnea-hypopnea and related clinical features in a population-based sample of subjects aged 30 to 70 yr. Am J Respir Crit Care Med 2001;163(3 Pt 1):685–9.

[7] Nieto FJ, Young TB, Lind BK, et al. Association of sleep-disordered breathing, sleep apnea, and hypertension in a large community-based study. Sleep Heart Health Study. JAMA 2000;283(14):1829–36.

[8] Lavie P, Herer P, Hoffstein V. Obstructive sleep apnoea syndrome as a risk factor for hypertension: population study. BMJ 2000;320(7233):479–82.

[9] Grote L, Ploch T, Heitmann J, et al. Sleep-related breathing disorder is an independent risk factor for systemic hypertension. Am J Respir Crit Care Med 1999;160(6):1875–82.

[10] Lavie P, Lavie L, Herer P. All-cause mortality in males with sleep apnoea syndrome: declining mortality rates with age. Eur Respir J 2005;25(3):514–20.

[11] Somers VK, Phil D, Dyken ME, et al. Sympathetic-nerve activity during sleep in normal subjects. N Engl J Med 1993;328(5):303–7.

[12] Hornyak M, Cejnar M, Elam M, et al. Sympathetic muscle nerve activity during sleep in man. Brain 1991;114:1281–95.

[13] Mancia G. Autonomic modulation of the cardiovascular system during sleep. N Engl J Med 1993; 328(5):347–9.

[14] Hedner J, Ejnell H, Sellgren J, et al. Is high and fluctuating muscle nerve sympathetic activity in the sleep apnoea syndrome of pathogenetic importance for the development of hypertension? J Hypertens Suppl 1988;6:S529–31.

[15] Somers VK, Dyken ME, Clary MP, et al. Sympathetic neural mechanisms in obstructive sleep apnea. J Clin Invest 1995;96(4):1897–904.

[16] Carlson JT, Hedner J, Elam M, et al. Augmented resting sympathetic activity in awake patients with obstructive sleep apnea. Chest 1993;103:1763–8.

[17] Heitmann J, Ehlenz K, Penzel T, et al. Sympathetic activity is reduced by nCPAP in hypertensive obstructive sleep apnoea patients. Eur Respir J 2004;23:255–62.

[18] Morgan BJ, Crabtree DC, Palta M, et al. Combined hypoxia and hypercapnia evokes long-lasting sympathetic activation in humans. J Appl Physiol 1995;79:205–13.

[19] Xie A, Skatrud JB, Crabtree DC, et al. Neurocirculatory consequences of intermittent asphyxia in humans. J Appl Physiol 2000;89(4):1333–9.

[20] Narkiewicz K, van de Borne PJ, Cooley RL, et al. Sympathetic activity in obese subjects with and without obstructive sleep apnea. Circulation 1998;98(8):772–6.

[21] Brooks D, Horner RL, Kozar LF, et al. Obstructive sleep apnea as a cause of systemic hypertension. Evidence from a canine model. J Clin Invest 1997;99(1):106–9.

[22] Ehlenz K. Regulation of blood volume-implications for cardiovascular pathophysiology in sleep apnoea. J Sleep Res 1995;4(S1):30–3.

[23] Krieger J, Follenius M, Sforza E, et al. Effects of treatment with nasal continuous positive airway pressure on atrial natriuretic peptide and arginine vasopressin release during sleep in patients with obstructive sleep apnoea. Clin Sci (Lond) 1991;80(5):443–9.

[24] Lavie L. Sleep apnea syndrome, endothelial dysfunction, and cardiovascular morbidity. Sleep 2004;27:1053–5.

[25] Ohike Y, Kozaki K, Iijima K, et al. Amelioration of vascular endothelial dysfunction in obstructive sleep apnea syndrome by nasal continuous positive airway pressure—possible involvement of nitric oxide and asymmetric NG, NG-dimethylarginine. Circ J 2005;69(2):221–6.

[26] Grote L, Kraiczi H, Hedner J. Reduced alpha- and beta(2)-adrenergic vascular response in patients with

with obstructive sleep apnea. Am J Respir Crit Care Med 2000;162(4 Pt 1):1480–7.

[27] Kraiczi H, Hedner J, Peker Y, et al. Increased vasoconstrictor sensitivity in obstructive sleep apnea. J Appl Physiol 2000;89(2):493–8.

[28] Schulz R. The vascular micromilieu in obstructive sleep apnoea. Eur Respir J 2005;25:780–2.

[29] Schulz R, Schmidt D, Blum A, et al. Decreased plasma levels of nitric oxide derivatives in obstructive sleep apnoea—response to CPAP therapy. Thorax 2000;55:1046–51.

[30] Engleman HM, Gough K, Martin SE, et al. Ambulatory blood pressure on and off continuous positive airway pressure therapy for the sleep apnea/hypopnea syndrome: effects in "non-dippers". Sleep 1996;19:378–81.

[31] Monasterio C, Vidal S, Duran J, et al. Effectiveness of continuous positive airway pressure in mild sleep apnea-hypopnea syndrome. Am J Respir Crit Care Med 2001;164:939–43.

[32] Dimsdale J, Loredo JS, Profant J. Effect of continuous positive airway pressure on blood pressure. A placebo trial. Hypertension 2000;35:144–7.

[33] Barnes M, Houston D, Worsnop CJ, et al. A randomized controlled trial of continuous positive airway pressure in mild obstructive sleep apnea. Am J Respir Crit Care Med 2002;165:773–80.

[34] Barbé F, Mayorolas LR, Duran J, et al. Treatment with continuous positive airway pressure is not effective in patients with sleep apnea but no daytime sleepiness. Ann Intern Med 2001;134:1015–23.

[35] Faccenda JF, Mackay TW, Boon NA, et al. Randomized placebo-controlled trial of continuous positive airway pressure on blood pressure in the sleep apnea-hypopnea syndrome. Am J Respir Crit Care Med 2001;163:334–48.

[36] Norman D, Loredo JS, Nelesen RA, et al. Effects of continuous positive airway pressure versus supplemental oxygen on 24-hour ambulatory blood pressure. Hypertension 2006;47(5):840–5.

[37] Pepperell JC, Ramdassingh-Dow S, Crosthwaite N, et al. Ambulatory blood pressure after therapeutic and subtherapeutic nasal continuous positive airway pressure for obstructive sleep apnoea: a randomised parallel trial. Lancet 2002;359:204–10.

[38] Mills PJ, Kennedy BP, Loredo JS, et al. Effects of nasal continuous positive airway pressure and oxygen supplementation on norepinephrine kinetics and cardiovascular responses in obstructive sleep apnea. J Appl Physiol 2006;100(1):343–8.

[39] Becker HF, Jerrentrup A, Ploch T, et al. Effect of nasal continuous positive airway pressure treatment on blood pressure in patients with obstructive sleep apnea. Circulation 2003;107:68–73.

[40] Logan AG, Tkacova R, Perlikowski SM, et al. Refractory hypertension and sleep apnoea: effect of CPAP on blood pressure and baroreflex. Eur Respir J 2003;21:241–7.

[41] Robinson GV, Smith DM, Langford BA, et al. Continuous positive airway pressure does not reduce blood pressure in nonsleepy hypertensive OSA patients. Eur Respir J 2006;27(6):1229–35.

[42] Rich S, editor. Primary pulmonary hypertension: executive summary from the world symposium on primary pulmonary hypertension. Geneva (Switzerland): World Health Organization; 1998.

[43] Marrone O, Bonsignore MR. Pulmonary hemodynamics in obstructive sleep apnoea. Sleep Med Rev 2002;6:175–93.

[44] Tilkian AG, Guillemina ult C, Schroeder JS, et al. Hemodynamics in sleep-induced apnea. Studies during wakefulness and sleep. Ann Intern Med 1976;85:714–9.

[45] Chaouat A, Weitzenblum E, Krieger J, et al. Pulmonary hemodynamics in the obstructive sleep apnea syndrome. Chest 1996;109:380–6.

[46] Laks L, Lehrhaft B, Grunstein RR, et al. Pulmonary hypertension in obstructive sleep apnea. Eur Respir J 1995;8:537–41.

[47] Sanner BM, Doberauer C, Konermann M, et al. Pulmonary arterial hypertension in patients with obstructive sleep apnea syndrome. Arch Intern Med 1997;157:2483–7.

[48] Arias M, Garcia-Rio F, Alonso-Fernandez A, et al. Pulmonary hypertension in obstructive sleep apnoea: effects of continuous positive airway pressure. Eur Respir J 2006;27:1106–13.

[49] Bady E, Achkar A, Pascal S, et al. Pulmonary arterial hypertension in patients with sleep apnea syndrome. Thorax 2000;55:934–9.

[50] Hender J, Enjell H, Caidahl K. Left ventricular hypetrophy independently of hypertension in patients with obstructive sleep apnea. J Hypertens 1990;8:941–6.

[51] Cargill JL, Kiely DG, Lipworth BJ. Adverse effects of hypoxemia on diastolic filling in humans. Clin Sci 1995;89:165–9.

[52] Podszus T, Bauer W, Mayer J, et al. Sleep apnea and pulmonary hypertension. Kin Wochenschr 1986;64:131–4.

[53] Bradley TD, Rutherford R, Grossman RF, et al. Role of daytime hypoxemia in the pathogenesis of right heart failure in the obstructive sleep apnea syndrome. Am Rev Respir Dis 1985;131:835–9.

[54] Motta J, Guilleminault C, Schroeder JS, et al. Tracheostomy and hemodynamic changes in sleep-induced apnea. Ann Intern Med 1978;89:454–8.

[55] Alchanatis M, Tourkohoriti G, Kakouros S, et al. Daytime pulmonary hypertension in patients with obstructive sleep apnea. Respiration 2001;68:566–72.

[56] Sajkov D, Wang T, Saunders NA, et al. Continuous positive airway pressure treatment improves pulmonary hemodynamics in patients with obstructive sleep apnea. Am J Respir Crit Care Med 2002;165:152–8.

[57] Sforza E, Krieger J, Weitzenblum E, et al. Long-term effects of treatment with nasal continuous positive airway pressure on daytime lung function and pulmonary hemodynamics in patients with obstructive sleep apnea. Am Rev Respir Dis 1990;141:866–70.

ELSEVIER SAUNDERS

SLEEP
MEDICINE
CLINICS

Sleep Med Clin 2 (2007) 559–564

Obstructive Sleep Apnea and Coronary Artery Disease

Jan Hedner, MD, PhD[a],*, Karl A. Franklin, MD, PhD[b],
Yüksel Peker, MD, PhD[a]

- Epidemiology
  Prevalence of OSA and CAD in the
    general population
  Prevalence of CAD in patients
    with OSA
- Prevalence of OSA in patients with CAD
  Incidence of CAD in longitudinal studies
- Pathogenesis
- Clinical course and prevention
- References

Epidemiologic studies suggest that obstructive sleep apnea (OSA) is over-represented in patients with coronary artery disease (CAD). Conversely, other studies have shown that the clinical course of CAD is initiated or accelerated by the presence of a coexisting sleep and breathing disorder. A rapidly evolving field of experimental data suggests that OSA, by mechanisms such as hypoxemia and reoxygenation, may trigger a sequence of events subsequently leading to development of atherosclerotic disease. However, it is reasonable to believe that the risk of developing vascular disease, and more specifically CAD—as a consequence of OSA—is influenced by several yet unidentified genotypic and phenotypic risk factors. Sleep apnea events induce a state of increased cardiac oxygen demand, but they are also frequently associated with low oxygen reserve because of lack of ventilation. This generates a situation where nocturnal angina can be triggered by the apnea in CAD patients. There is growing evidence that elimination of sleep apnea benefits patients with OSA at risk of CAD in the immediate and long term.

Epidemiology

The risk of experiencing angina pectoris or an acute coronary syndrome, such as unstable angina, acute myocardial infarction (MI), or sudden cardiac death appears to be increased during the late hours of sleep or in the early morning hours after awakening [1]. Early speculation was that this circadian distribution is in part explained by obstructive breathing. A recent registry study of a sleep laboratory cohort demonstrated that OSA patients had a peak in sudden death from cardiac cause during the sleeping hours (midnight to 6 AM) which contrasted with the nadir of sudden death from cardiac cause in those without OSA or the general population [2]. The epidemiologic support for a causal relationship between OSA and CAD is rapidly increasing but firm evidence from randomized controlled trials is still lacking. The relationship between OSA and CAD is generally stronger in clinical cohorts than in studies dealing with the general population. This discrepancy may be explained by the fact that patients participating in clinical cohort

---

a Department of Pulmonary Medicine, Sahlgrenska University Hospital, SE-413 45 Gothenburg, Sweden
b Department of Pulmonary Medicine, Norrland University Hospital, SE-901 85 Umeå, Sweden
* Corresponding author.
E-mail address: jan.hedner@lungall.gu.se (J. Hedner).

1556-407X/07/$ – see front matter © 2007 Elsevier Inc. All rights reserved.
sleep.theclinics.com

doi:10.1016/j.jsmc.2007.07.008

[21] Mooe T, Franklin KA, Wiklund U, et al. Sleep-disordered breathing in patients with coronary artery disease. Chest 2000;117:1597–602.

[22] Moruzzi P, Sarzi-Braga S, Rossi M, et al. Sleep apnoea in ischaemic heart disease: differences between acute and chronic coronary syndromes. Heart 1999;82:343–7.

[23] Sanner BM, Konermann M, Doberauer C, et al. Sleep-disordered breathing in patients referred for angina evaluation—association with left ventricular dysfunction. Clin Cardiol 2001;24:146–50.

[24] Takama N, Kurabayashi M. Possibility of close relationship between sleep disordered breathing and acute coronary syndrome. J Cardiol 2007;49: 171–7.

[25] Zaninelli A, Fariello R, Boni E, et al. Snoring and risk of cardiovascular disease. Int J Cardiol 1991; 32:347–52.

[26] Jennum P, Hein HO, Suadicani P, et al. Risk of ischemic heart disease in self-reported snorers. A prospective study of 2,937 men aged 54 to 74 years: the Copenhagen male study. Chest 1995;108:138–42.

[27] Zamarron C, Gude F, Otero Otero Y, et al. Snoring and myocardial infarction: a 4-year follow-up study. Respir Med 1999;93:108–12.

[28] Lindberg E, Janson C, Svärdsudd K, et al. Increased mortality among sleepy snorers: a prospective population based study. Thorax 1998; 53:631–7.

[29] Peker Y, Norum J, Hedner J, et al. Increased incidence of coronary artery disease in obstructive sleep apnoea: a seven-year follow-up [abstract]. Eur Respir J 2001;18(Suppl 33):518s.

[30] Peker Y, Hedner J, Norum J, et al. Increased incidence of cardiovascular disease in middle-aged men with obstructive sleep apnea: a seven-year follow-up. Am J Respir Crit Care 2002;166:159–65.

[31] Marin JM, Carrizo SJ, Vicente E, et al. Long-term cardiovascular outcome in men with obstructive sleep apnoea-hypopnoea with or without treatment with continuous positive airway pressure: an observational study. Lancet 2005;365: 1046–53.

[32] Andreas S, Schulz R, Werner GS, et al. Prevalence of obstructive sleep apnoea in patients with coronary artery disease. Coron Artery Dis 1996;7: 541–5.

[33] Hedner J, Ejnell H, Sellgren J, et al. Is high and fluctuating muscle nerve sympathetic activity in the sleep apnoea syndrome of pathogenetic importance for the development of hypertension? J Hypertens 1988;6(Suppl 4):529–31.

[34] Parati G, Di Rienzo M, Bonsignore MR, et al. Autonomic cardiac regulation in obstructive sleep apnea syndrome: evidence from spontaneous baroreflex analysis during sleep. J Hypertens 1997;15(12 Pt 2):1621–6.

[35] Ryan S, Ward S, Heneghan C, et al. Predictors of decreased spontaneous baroreflex sensitivity in obstructive sleep apnea syndrome. Chest 2007; 131:1100–7.

[36] Kraiczi H, Hedner J, Peker Y, et al. Increased vasoconstrictor sensitivity in obstructive sleep apnea. J Appl Physiol 2000;89:493–8.

[37] Carlson JT, Rangemark C, Hedner JA. Attenuated endothelium-dependent vascular relaxation in patients with sleep apnea. J Hypertens 1996; 14:577–84.

[38] Narkiewicz K, Somers VK. Sympathetic nerve activity in obstructive sleep apnoea. Acta Physiol Scand 2003;177:385–90.

[39] Schulz R, Mahmoudi S, Hattar K, et al. Enhanced release of superoxide from polymorphonuclear neutrophils in obstructive sleep apnea. Impact of continuous positive airway pressure therapy. Am J Respir Crit Care Med 2000;162:566–70.

[40] Lavie L. Obstructive sleep apnoea syndrome—an oxidative stress disorder. Sleep Med Rev 2003;7: 35–51.

[41] Lavie L, Kraiczi H, Hefetz A, et al. Plasma vascular endothelial growth factor in sleep apnea syndrome: effects of nasal continuous positive air pressure treatment. Am J Respir Crit Care Med 2002;165:1624–8.

[42] Yokoe T, Minoguchi K, Matsuo H, et al. Elevated levels of C-reactive protein and interleukin-6 in patients with obstructive sleep apnea syndrome are decreased by nasal continuous positive airway pressure. Circulation 2003;107: 1129–34.

[43] Ohga E, Tomita T, Wada H, et al. Effects of obstructive sleep apnea on circulating ICAM-1, IL-8, and MCP-1. J Appl Physiol 2003;94:179–84.

[44] Ryan S, Taylor CT, McNicholas WT. Selective activation of inflammatory pathways by intermittent hypoxia in obstructive sleep apnea syndrome. Circulation 2005;112:2660–7.

[45] Dyugovskaya L, Lavie P, Lavie L. Phenotypic and functional characterization of blood gammadelta T cells in sleep apnea. Am J Respir Crit Care Med 2003;168:242–9.

[46] El-Solh AA, Mador MJ, Sikka P, et al. Adhesion molecules in patients with coronary artery disease and moderate-to-severe obstructive sleep apnea. Chest 2002;121:1541–7.

[47] Libby P. Atherosclerosis: the new view. Sci Am 2002;286:46–55.

[48] Peker Y, Hedner J, Kraiczi H, et al. Respiratory disturbance index: an independent predictor of mortality in coronary artery disease. Am J Respir Crit Care Med 2000;162:81–6.

[49] Mooe T, Franklin KA, Holmström K, et al. Sleep-disordered breathing and coronary artery disease: long-term prognosis. Am J Respir Crit Care Med 2001;164:1910–3.

[50] Hagenah GC, Gueven E, Andreas S. Influence of obstructive sleep apnea in coronary artery disease: A 10-year follow-up. Respir Med 2006;100: 180–2.

[51] Schafer H, Koehler U, Ploch T, et al. Sleep-related myocardial ischemia and sleep structure in patients with obstructive sleep apnea and coronary heart disease. Chest 1997;111:387–93.

SLEEP MEDICINE CLINICS

Sleep Med Clin 2 (2007) 565–574

ELSEVIER SAUNDERS

Obstructive Sleep Apnea and Left Ventricular Systolic and Diastolic Dysfunction

Francisco García-Río, MD, PhD[a,b,]*, Miguel A. Arias, MD, PhD[c]

- Epidemiologic data
- Physiopathologic mechanisms
- Sistolic dysfunction in OSA
- Diastolic dysfunction in OSA
- Clinical impact
- The effect of CPAP
- References

The accumulating evidence of associations between cardiovascular complications and obstructive sleep apnea (OSA) has had an undeniable impact on attitudes toward this condition. Beyond the well-recognized relationship between OSA and arterial hypertension, there have been many publications in recent years with evidence regarding connections between OSA and left ventricular dysfunction, both diastolic and systolic, with or without heart failure.

The conditions of OSA and left ventricular dysfunction are very prevalent [1,2] and have notable sociosanitary impacts because of their mortality and associated costs. Nevertheless, their relationship is still not entirely clear, not only regarding clinical and therapeutic implications, but also with regard to the pathophysiologic mechanisms involved and the epidemiology of the phenomenon. This is due, among other causes, to the small sample sizes in the studies published, the types of sleep registers used, conceptual differences between

investigators, and the existence of confounding factors such as obesity, arterial hypertension, hypoxemia, and daytime hypercapnia or airflow limitation.

This article reviews epidemiologic data that potentially implicates OSA syndrome as a cause of left ventricular systolic and diastolic dysfunction, as well as the possible pathophysiologic mechanisms involved. The clinical implications of this relationship is also considered, and the available data regarding the efficacy of continuous positive airway pressure therapy (CPAP) in patients with OSA and left ventricular dysfunction will be reviewed.

Epidemiologic data

Various data suggest that OSA is more frequent in patients with heart failure than in patients without this condition. The mean values in the main studies published [3–7] show the frequency of OSA in patients with heart failure ranging between 11% to

This work was supported by Grants No. 01/0278 from the Fondo de Investigación Sanitaria and No. 2000 from Neumomadrid.
[a] Hospital Universitario La Paz, Alfredo Marquerie 11, izqda, 1° A, 28034-Madrid, Spain
[b] School of Medicine, Universidad Autónoma de Madrid, Arzobispo Morcillo s/n, 28046-Madrid, Spain
[c] Cardiology Department, Hospital Virgen de la Salud, Avenida de Europa 3, Esc. 2, 3° C, 45005-Toledo, Spain
* Corresponding author. Hospital Universitario La Paz, Alfredo Marquerie 11, izqda, 1° A, 28034-Madrid, Spain
E-mail address: fgr01m@gmail.com (F. García-Río).

doi:10.1016/j.jsmc.2007.07.006
sleep.theclinics.com

38%, which is greater than that described in the general population [2]. The differences seen between the aforementioned studies may be explained by their different values for the apnea-hypopnea index (AHI), as well as the variability in the definitions of hypopnea used. Some investigators considered hypopnea to be a decrease of 2% in oxygen saturation (SaO_2) [8], while others preferred a 4% decrease or the presence of arousal from sleep [5].

The principal prospective study cited above [5] included 81 men with stable systolic heart failure (left ventricular ejection fraction—or LVEF—less than 45%), in a polysomnographic study, taking AHI greater than or equal to 15 h^{-1} as a threshold. Of all the subjects, 41 (51%) presented moderate to high AHI during sleep, with a mean of 44 ± 19 h^{-1}. Some 11% of the subjects studied presented OSAS, while 40% had central apneas. Of the 41 subjects with respiratory dysfunction during sleep, the prevalence of atrial fibrillation and ventricular arrhythmias was also significantly higher than in the other subjects.

A large retrospective study [7] included 450 subjects of both genders (382 men, 68 women) with systolic heart failure and a mean LVEF of $27 \pm 16\%$. Of these, 61% had an AHI greater or equal to 15 h^{-1}, greater than the 51% reported in the Javaheri and colleagues [5] prospective study mentioned above. Of the 450 subjects, 168 (37.3%) presented OSA, with a greater prevalence in men (38%) than in women (31%). The differences in OSA prevalence seen between this study and that of Javaheri and colleagues [5] could be a result of the subjects in the former being referred to a sleep laboratory because they presented OSA risk factors, which was not the case in the second study. Nevertheless, it is significant that OSA prevalence in these study populations was greater than that seen in healthy subjects [2].

In a larger series of patients with systolic heart failure, OSA was present in 12% of the cases [9]. Unlike central sleep apnea syndrome with Cheyne-Stokes respiration (CSA-CSR), OSA is more frequently seen in obese patients with heart failure who snore habitually [9]. These risk factors of OSA in patients with heart failure are similar to those of OSA without heart failure. Prevalence of sleep apnea is also increased in patients with mild systolic dysfunction. Vazir and colleagues [10] have recently described a 15% OSA incidence rate in men with heart failure caused by mild left ventricular systolic dysfunction.

There are also few studies in which the prevalence of OSA in patients with isolated left ventricular diastolic dysfunction has been evaluated. Taking an AHI greater or equal to 10 h^{-1} as pathologic,

Chan and colleagues [11] determined the prevalence of OSA in 20 patients of both genders with isolated symptomatic diastolic dysfunction, evaluated using echocardiography, and found that 11 patients (55%) suffered respiratory disorders during sleep. Seven (35% of the sample) had OSA and four (20%) had central apneas. The patients with and without respiratory disorders were comparable with regards to arterial pressure, $PaCO_2$, and body mass index (BMI). Large scale epidemiologic studies will be necessary to clarify the real prevalence of sleep apnea disorders in patients with isolated left ventricular diastolic dysfunction because it has been shown that a large proportion of older patients with heart failure present isolated diastolic dysfunction [12], and sleep respiratory disorders may be prevalent in this patient population.

On the other hand, the appearance of acute nocturnal pulmonary edema has been described in some patients with OSA and normal left ventricular function [13]. This also refers to the fact that normotensive patients with OSA have thicker left ventricular (LV) walls than healthy subjects [14]. In another study, left ventricular hypertrophy was identified in 41% of subjects with OSA, hypertrophy was directly correlated with AHI and sleep time with SaO_2 less than 90% [15]. Improvement of systolic and diastolic function of the LV, when obstructive apneas are eliminated with CPAP, reinforces the relationship between the two disorders [16–20].

The Sleep Heart Health Study [6], the largest epidemiological study (with 6,424 subjects) analyzed the association between OSA and various cardiovascular disorders. This study reported that AHI greater than or equal to 11 h^{-1} increased the risk of congestive heart failure 2.38 times (92% confidence interval 1.22–4.62), independent of other factors. The physiopathologic connections between heart failure and OSA makes it more clear how, in individuals with heart failure from any cause, the development of OSA will favor the progression of heart failure by various mechanisms, ultimately reaching the most severe stage [1], with all the unfavorable clinical, therapeutic, and prognostic implications that entails.

Physiopathologic mechanisms

Obstructive apneas-hypopneas have immediate hemodynamic repercussions and establish mid- to long-term changes (Table 1) that facilitate the development of left ventricular dysfunction. In acute form, the drop in intrathoracic pressure during obstructive apneas increases the afterload, which is determined by the left ventricular transmural pressure. This is derived by subtracting the

Table 1: Mechanisms implicated in mid- to long-term development of left ventricular dysfunction in patients with OSA

Mechanism	Alterations
Hemodynamic	Systemic hypertension Cardiac myocyte necrosis β-adrenoceptor desensitivization Cardiac arrhythmias
Neurohumoral	Increased sympathetic activity Reduced parasympathetic modulation
Inflammatory and oxidative stress	Increased IL-6, CRP and TNF-α Increased oxygen free radicals
Endothelial dysfunction	Impaired endothelial mediated vasodilatation Increased endothelin, ICAM-1, VCAM-1, and adhesion of leukocytes to endothelium
Prothrombotic	Increased plasminogen, activator inhibitor, platelet activity and aggregation

Abbreviations: CRP, C-reactive protein; ICAM-1, intercellular adhesion molecule; IL-6, interleukin-6; TNF-α, tumor necrosis factor-α; VCAM, vascular cell adhesion molecule.

intrathoracic pressure from the LV end-systolic pressure [21–23].

In the longer term, the succession of ineffective inspiratory efforts against the occluded upper airway during obstructive apnea, with the concomitant increase in the LV afterload, favors the development of concentric compensatory hypertrophy, with greater oxygen demand and consumption on the part of the LV myocardium [24]. The continued repetition of these parietal ventricular stress episodes may induce the activation of genes involved in ventricular remodeling, and give rise to variable degrees of contractile dysfunction [25]. Furthermore, the excessive negative intrathoracic pressure during apneas may cause an alteration in LV relaxation properties, complicating the process of ventricular filling in the diastole [26]. Left ventricular filling may also be impaired because of leftward septal displacement caused by right ventricular volume overload during OSA [27].

Hypoxemia secondary to apneas and hypopneas can affect the cardiovascular system through various mechanisms, such as a decrease in oxygen transported to the myocardium, an increase in the activity of the sympathetic nervous system, the development of endothelial dysfunction, and fostering a procoagulant state (for review see Ref. [28]).

Animal models have shown that chronic exposition to an intermittent hypoxic model induces an increase in arterial pressure, end-diastolic pressure of the left ventricle and of the LV mass, as well as a decrease in cardiac output, left ventricular shortening fraction, and LVEF [29]. This demonstrates that chronic intermittent hypoxia contributes to the development of ventricular hypertrophy, distention, and dysfunction. Hypoxemia causes a decrease in the liberation of oxygen to the myocardium, an effect that is magnified in those patients with limited blood flow because of the presence of atherosclerotic obstructive coronary lesions. The hypocapnia that may present secondary to hyperventilation after apnea or hypopneas can decrease oxygen liberation to the myocardium, because of both coronary vasoconstriction [30] as well as deviation of the hemoglobin saturation curve to the left. This lower transmission of myocardial oxygen can affect the systolic and diastolic function of the left ventricle.

Hypoxemia also causes increases in sympathetic activity and systemic arterial pressure [31,32]. In addition, it produces a reduction in sustained vagal tone in patients with OSA [33]. Both circumstances favor an increase in the myocardial consumption of oxygen when under increased demand.

There is still no direct, conclusive evidence that demonstrates that OSA can cause atherosclerosis. However, intermittent hypoxemia caused by apneas, followed by postapnea reoxygenation, probably contributes to the generation of oxygen free radicals and certain cellular adhesion molecules [34,35]. After chronic exposition to intermittent hypoxia, increases in LV myocardial lipid peroxides and decreases in levels of LV myocardial superoxide dismutase have been reported [29]. It is possible that intermittent hypoxia produces oxidative stress similar to the classic model of myocardial ischemia-reperfusion injury, and because of an increase in sympathoadrenal tone [36]. Definitively, it appears that the development of systolic LV dysfunction is time dependent and associated with an increase in oxidative stress of the myocardial fibers, as well as a decrease in antioxidant activity. Furthermore, there is a relationship between the degree of oxidative stress and the severity of LV dysfunction [29,36].

The phenomenon of an indirect lesion may originate from leukocyte activation and the generation of an endothelial vascular response, favoring endothelial dysfunction, as well as setting in motion atherosclerotic processes. It has also been demonstrated that hypoxemia can induce apoptosis in cardiac and endothelial cells [37,38], as well as induce the expression of specific genes implicated in regulating the synthesis of endothelial vasodilators, such as nitric oxide [39], the plasma concentration of which has been found to be reduced in patients with OSA [40]. Decreased vasodilator response has been reported in subjects with OSA, which improves with CPAP treatment, in direct relation with the decrease in sympathetic activity caused by CPAP [41].

Various procoagulant effects have been reported in OSA subjects, such as the increase in platelet activation [42] and an increase in levels of fibrinogen or factor VII coagulant activation, all of which can be attenuated with CPAP treatment. Subjects with OSA have elevated levels of C-reactive protein in relation to controls of similar age, gender, and BMI. These elevations are proportional to AHI [43].

Hemodynamic changes produced during obstructive apneas may potentially facilitate or augment the liberation of B-type natriuretic peptide [44]. Preliminary data suggest that patients with OSA without overt heart failure presented higher levels of this peptide at night, in direct relation to elevations in levels of arterial pressure and the duration of the apneas [45].

Finally, arousals that are produced at the end of apneas, together with hypoxemia, also increase sympathetic activity and decrease vagal tone [46,47]. The repetition of arousals increases the consumption of oxygen, favoring LV hypertrophy and promoting myocardial remodeling.

At this point, there is limited information available about which of the mechanisms described here has the most relevant role in the pathophysiology of LV dysfunction in OSA patients. It is possible that each patient establishes their own balance between the different factors. It has been shown, for example, that during the recovery period for obstructive apneas during nonrapid eye movement sleep, there is an intense reduction in systolic volume, coinciding with an increase in arterial pressure and a slight increase in heart rate that does not prevent a decrease in cardiac output [48]. These findings would attribute a large portion of the deterioration of LV function to an increase in the afterload, which appears to be related to the sympathetic discharge produced by arousals [48].

The process of ventricular remodeling is essential as the final common pathway to the distinct factors implicated in the effect of apneas and hypopneas on LV function. This process has a fundamental role in hypertrophy, loss of myocytes, and excessive interstitial fibrosis [49,50].

Fundamentally, the pathophysiologic mechanisms involved in OSA and heart failure syndrome converge at two principal points, which can facilitate the progression of ventricular failure. On the one hand, there are the deleterious effects of the overactivation of the sympathetic nervous system and the general inhibition of the cardiovascular system by the parasympathetic nervous system. On the other hand, there are the alterations in left ventricular preload and afterload, and the effects of hypoxemia, especially in the left ventricle, with dysfunction caused by any type of heart disease. Some of the consequences of sympathetic overactivity on this already altered ventricular myocardium include necrosis and myocyte apoptosis, loss of sensitivity and down-regulation of the β-adrenergic receptors, arrhythmogenesis, and an increase in mortality [51–53]. The stimulation of the renal sympathetic nerve terminals causes the activation of the renin-angiotensin-aldosterone system, which provokes a greater retention of sodium and an increase in volemia [52], with the consequent negative effects on myocardial performance.

Verdecchia and colleagues [54] report on the greater influence of systemic arterial hypertension (HT) on the development of left ventricular hypertrophy when the former is during sleep, rather than wakefulness. The highest figures for nocturnal arterial pressure are produced in patients with HT and OSA, with respect to subjects with HT and without OSA, situating the former at greater risk of developing left ventricular hypertrophy [55].

Dogs subjected to repeated apneas over a period of weeks developed nocturnal and diurnal HT [56], LV hypertrophy, LV systolic dysfunction, and interstitial pulmonary edema [57]. Given that the cardiac output in patients with LV dysfunction is especially sensitive to an increase in the afterload, the most direct mechanism by which OSA can degrade left ventricular function would be its effect on systemic arterial pressure. When a patient with heart failure suffers repeated obstructive apneas, arterial pressure is raised to levels greater than those seen during the day [58]. In patients with stable heart failure under medical treatment, the presence of OSA is associated with increases in daytime arterial pressure proportional to the number of apneas and hypopneas [59].

Repeated increases in negative intrathoracic pressure that are produced during obstructive sleep apneas, which can reach pressures up to −65 mm Hg [19] in patients with heart failure, suppose a large increase in the afterload and myocardial oxygen demand. In patients with heart failure, this results in a greater reduction in systolic volume than in control subjects with preserved ventricular function [60]. The repetition of these events up to hundreds of times a night represents an important stress on the ventricular myocardium, which can set in motion the mechanisms implicated in ventricular remodeling, with a more compromised ventricular function in the long term [25].

Finally, the elevated levels of inflammatory mediators in subjects with OSA, O_2 radical production, and the development of varying degrees of endothelial dysfunction can also promote and accelerate the process of atherosclerosis [34,35,43,61,62]. Given that ischemic heart disease is the principle cause of left ventricular dysfunction, OSA can worsen this dysfunction and its effects on the coronary arteries.

Sistolic dysfunction in OSA

Despite the pathophysiologic mechanisms that indicate an influence of OSA on systolic function of the LV, various cross-sectional studies have reported normal LVEF in patients with OSA, identical to that of normal subjects without OSA [14,63–65]. Nevertheless, the interpretation of these preliminary studies may be problematic because their findings are based on small patient samples, they evaluate left ventricular systolic function in a heterogeneous manner (echocardiography, radionucleotide ventriculography, and so forth) and they do not control for possible coadjuvant factors such as hypoxemia, hypercapnia, and systemic arterial pressure.

A canine model has contributed valuable information regarding the repercussion of OSA on the left ventricular systolic function by verifying that, after 1 to 3 months of simulated obstructive apneas, a decrease in LVEF on two-dimensional echocardiography is induced [22].

In a study with 169 consecutive subjects diagnosed with OSA and without known heart disease, Laaban and colleagues [66] identified, by means of radionucleotide ventriculography, that 7.7% had left ventricular systolic dysfunction (LVEF less than 50%). They also tested that this systolic dysfunction was not related to age, BMI, AHI, nocturnal oxygenation, or HT. It is very unlikely that LV systolic dysfunction was caused by silent coronary artery disease, given that segmental left ventricular wall motion abnormalities were not demonstrated by radionuclide angiography or echocardiography [66].

With the goal of evaluating left ventricular systolic function in patients with OSA as early as possible, the authors analyzed the cardiovascular response to progressive exercise of 31 normotensive patients with OSA, but without clinical heart failure, and with normal resting LVEF [67]. Stroke volume was determined during the exercise using a carbon dioxide (CO_2) rebreathing technique [68]. With respect to the control group, the patients with OSA presented reduced cardiac output and systolic volume responses during exercise [67].

Diastolic dysfunction in OSA

In a small series of patients with diastolic heart failure (normal LVEF), Chan and colleagues [11] determined that 55% had associated OSA and found a relationship between the degree of nocturnal hypoxemia and left ventricular diastolic dysfunction.

Shortly thereafter, Alchanatis and colleagues [63] compared left ventricular function in 15 patients with OSA to 11 obese patients without OSA. With respect to the latter, the patients with OSA had left ventricular diastolic dysfunction, but not systolic dysfunction. In a larger series, Fung and colleagues [69] identified up to 37% of patients with OSA that showed a pattern of impaired relaxation of the LV, a mild grade of diastolic dysfunction. In obese patients pending gastric bypass surgery with moderate to severe OSA, a greater incidence of left ventricular diastolic dysfunction has been described, reaching 50% in patients when evaluated by Doppler and tissue-Doppler echocardiography [70].

Recently, in 14 patients with OSA and 14 control subjects, Kasikcioglu and colleagues [71] determined that patients with OSA had a higher aortic stiffness index and a lower aortic distensibility index, as well a lower peak velocity of myocardial systolic and diastolic waves. This finding brought forth the hypothesis that OSA may affect the elastic properties of the ascending aorta, because of increased sympathetic stimulation or direct vascular effect (acute hypoxic stress), which would favor left ventricular diastolic dysfunction. In fact, under normal conditions, the aortic diameter decreases because the diastole acts as a pump generator. Following these general lines of argument, the increase in aortic rigidity increases the left ventricular afterload, which worsens myocardial perfusion and induces changes in the properties of the myocytes and interstices, possibly favoring the development of left ventricular diastolic dysfunction [71].

In patients with OSA, it is possible that left ventricular diastolic dysfunction occurs earlier than systolic dysfunction. In fact, in a prospective study, the incidence of diastolic dysfunction was studied in 15 healthy subjects and 27 middle-aged subjects recently diagnosed with OSA, without heart failure, HT, or other known risk factors for diastolic dysfunction [17]. Left ventricular diastolic dysfunction was identified in 15 of the 27 subjects with OSA (55%) and only 3 of the 15 control subjects (20%) ($P = 0.02$), this being in the more common pattern of impaired relaxation, which typifies milder degrees of left ventricular diastolic dysfunction [17].

Similar findings have also been reported in children with OSA and without known heart disease [72]. No alterations in left ventricular systolic function were identified in these subjects, yet the investigators showed evidence of diastolic dysfunction directly related to AHI, and independent of obesity, arterial pressure, and left ventricular mass [72].

The importance of the development of diastolic dysfunction stems from two facts. First, the proportion of patients with heart failure that present normal left ventricular systolic function is elevated, thus alterations in diastolic function in these patients are the fundamental pathophysiologic axis. Second, patients with diastolic heart failure present a prognosis similar to that of patients with systolic heart failure, with elevated mortality during follow-up [73].

Clinical impact

The hypothesis that OSA contributes to the development of heart failure by altering left ventricular systolic and diastolic function took on force when reviewing the available data. It has been speculated that OSA might have a relevant role in the pathogenesis of left ventricular failure in specific patients with heart failure of unknown origin, and that OSA could be a causal agent independent of heart failure. The pathophysiologic mechanisms that are put in motion during repeated episodes of apneas and hypopneas, and which implicate the cardiovascular system, facilitate the progression of heart failure from other causes, to which these respiratory events during sleep are later added, either as a consequence of or independently of heart failure.

It is possible that heart failure can contribute to the development of OSA, in addition to causing CSA-CSR. In fact, the presence of CSA-CSR can destabilize the upper airway and predispose it to collapse by reducing the dilatory muscular tone of the pharynx, secondary to the loss of respiratory drive in the apnea phases. Furthermore, the retention of liquid that accompanies congestive heart failure may cause adoption of the supine decubitus position during sleep, to produce edema of the soft tissues of the throat and pharynx, which can narrow the upper airway and even cause its intermittent collapse [74].

The clinical characteristics of OSA in patients with heart failure are similar to those of other patients with OSA and normal ventricular function. As such, they often represent obese patients with a history of regular snoring. Nevertheless, the typical excessive daytime sleepiness of OSA is only present in a smaller portion of these patients [5,75], which suggests that many patients with heart failure may have undiagnosed OSA.

OSA may have a particularly negative effect on subjects with left ventricular dysfunction, given that the afterload increase derived from the obstructive apneas falls much more heavily on the ventricle whose function is already altered than on the ventricle that still conserves its functionality [76]. Therefore, when a subject with left ventricular dysfunction is submitted to important negative intrathoracic pressure during the Müller maneuver, they experience important drops in systolic volume and cardiac output, which take longer to recover from in the postapneic period than in subjects with normal ventricular function [60]. Furthermore, the increase in sympathetic activity produced in OSA [77–79] has very adverse prognostic effects on patients with coexisting ventricular dysfunction.

Very recently, a large series of 700 subjects was described with heart failure (New York Heart Association greater than or equal to II and LVEF less than or equal to 40%) and in optimal medical treatment, of which 36% had OSA [80]. In relation with CSA-CSR, the patients with OSA appear to be less symptomatic, have a greater LVEF, and a greater exercise tolerance, estimated by the peak oxygen uptake and by the distance walked in the 6-minute walk test [80].

The effect of CPAP

There are a number of studies [81–83] on the effect of CPAP on hypertension, which are discussed elsewhere in this volume. There are numerous data about the effect of CPAP on ventricular dysfunction in patients without heart failure. Kreiger and colleagues [84] showed that one year of treatment with CPAP increased LVEF in patients who had severe OSA, no ischemic heart disease, and a basal LVEF greater than 50%. In normotensive subjects with OSA and without overt heart failure, it has been shown that 3 months of treatment with CPAP were able to improve cardiac output and systolic volume responses during exercise [67]. Nevertheless, it has still not been possible to clarify whether this improved left ventricular systolic function is due to an increase in the preload (by improving diastolic function), a reduction in the afterload, or a direct increase in cardiac contractility.

Other studies analyzed the effects of CPAP treatment on left ventricular diastolic dysfunction in patients with OSA [16,17,20,63]. In all of these, the objective was an improvement in functional diastolic parameters after CPAP treatment. Arias and colleagues [17] conducted a prospective study, randomized and controlled with placebo (sham CPAP), which evaluated the effect of 3 months of CPAP treatment on standard echocardiographic parameters of diastolic function in 27 subjects with

OSA, but without heart failure. CPAP improved all the diastolic ventricular parameters analyzed [17]. In children, a year of treatment has also been shown to achieve significant improvements in left ventricular diastolic function [72].

The most recent information available on the application of CPAP in patients with heart failure and OSA is still limited, although the majority of studies indicate that this treatment has a favorable clinical effect on multiple structural and functional parameters of the cardiovascular system [17–20,85,86]. Some of the beneficial effects of CPAP in these patients are: the reduction of sympathetic nervous system activity during sleep as well as wakefulness [79,87], an increase in heart rate variability [33], improved endothelial vasodilatation capacity, hypercoagulation, and leukocyte activation [35,40,42,88]. Furthermore, the elimination of apneas and hypopneas with CPAP prevents recurrent hypoxemia, reduces nocturnal arterial pressure and heart rate, and increases baroreflex sensitivity [89]. The suppression of obstructive apneas and arousals causes a reduction in myocardial oxygen demand by reducing sympathetic activity, increasing intrathoracic pressure, and reducing left ventricular end-diastolic pressure. Furthermore, suppression increases coronary flow by increasing cardiac output, and therefore, coronary perfusion pressure [90]. The effect on the resulting systolic volume depends on left ventricular function. When it is normal, the application of CPAP reduces venous return, limits ventricular filling, lowers the preload, and reduces systolic volume. To the contrary, when ventricular function is altered and left ventricular end-diastolic pressure is therefore elevated, the reduction in the preload improves the properties of the myocardial tension-length and increases the systolic volume of the cardiac output [90]. Apart from this, it is also important to mention that there is no evidence that demonstrates that regular pharmacologic treatment for heart failure positively influences OSA severity [91].

Meanwhile, similar to the therapeutic effects of CPAP in patients with OSA and without heart failure, acute titration with CPAP in patients with systolic heart failure has been shown to eliminate OSA [92]. Furthermore, chronic application of CPAP (1–3 months) increases left ventricular ejection fraction [18,86]. Kaneko and colleagues [18] conducted a randomized, controlled study to evaluate the effect of 1 month of CPAP treatment. It included 24 subjects with heart failure caused by ischemic and nonischemic dilated cardiomyopathy, and OSA (AHI greater than or equal to 20 h^{-1}). Subjects were receiving optimized pharmacologic treatment for heart failure (including β-blockers in 50% of the patients) and had been clinically stable for the 3 previous months. In the 12 subjects under CPAP treatment, a reduction in daytime heart rate (68 ± 3 versus 64 ± 3 beats per minute, $P = 0.007$) and systolic arterial pressure (126 ± 6 versus 116 ± 5 mm Hg, $P = 0.020$) was found, as well as a 9% increase in mean LVEF (25 ± 3 versus 34 ± 2%, $P < 0.001$).

The largest study to date, Mansfield and colleagues [86] examined the effects of three months of CPAP treatment in 40 subjects with systolic heart failure and OSA (mean AHI 25 h^{-1} and mean LVEF 38%). After the 3 months of CPAP treatment, an increase in LVEF (38 ± 3% versus 43 ± 0%, $P = 0.04$) was seen, together with an improvement in quality of life questionnaires and daytime sleepiness, as well as a decrease in nighttime urinary catecholamine levels. The lesser magnitude of LVEF increase in the Mansfield (5%) group with respect to Kaneko (9%) could be a result of a reduced effect on the afterload. In fact, in the Mansfield and colleagues [86] study, CPAP was unable to reduce measures of systemic arterial pressure.

There is still no relevant information on the long-term benefits of CPAP treatment in patients with OSA and the effects on morbidity and mortality remain to be determined.

References

[1] Hunt SA. ACC/AHA 2005 guideline update for the diagnosis and management of chronic heart failure in the adult: a report of the American College of Cardiology/American Heart Association Task Force on Practice Guidelines (Writing Committee to Update the 2001 Guidelines for the Evaluation and Management of Heart Failure). J Am Coll Cardiol 2005;46(6):e1–82.

[2] Young T, Palta M, Dempsey J, et al. The occurrence of sleep-disordered breathing among middle-aged adults. N Engl J Med 1993;328(17): 1230–5.

[3] Bradley TD, Floras JS. Sleep apnea and heart failure: Part I: obstructive sleep apnea. Circulation 2003;107(12):1671–8.

[4] Javaheri S, Parker TJ, Wexler L, et al. Occult sleep-disordered breathing in stable congestive heart failure. Ann Intern Med 1995;122(7):487–92.

[5] Javaheri S, Parker TJ, Liming JD, et al. Sleep apnea in 81 ambulatory male patients with stable heart failure. Types and their prevalences, consequences, and presentations. Circulation 1998; 97(21):2154–9.

[6] Shahar E, Whitney CW, Redline S, et al. Sleep-disordered breathing and cardiovascular disease: cross-sectional results of the Sleep Heart Health Study. Am J Respir Crit Care Med 2001;163(1): 19–25.

[7] Sin DD, Fitzgerald F, Parker JD, et al. Risk factors for central and obstructive sleep apnea in 450

men and women with congestive heart failure. Am J Respir Crit Care Med 1999;160(4):1101–6.

[8] Lanfranchi PA, Braghiroli A, Bosimini E, et al. Prognostic value of nocturnal Cheyne-Stokes respiration in chronic heart failure. Circulation 1999;99(11):1435–40.

[9] Javaheri S. Sleep disorders in systolic heart failure: a prospective study of 100 male patients. The final report. Int J Cardiol 2006;106(1):21–8.

[10] Vasan A, Hastings PC, Dayer M, et al. A high prevalence of sleep disordered breathing in men with mild symptomatic chronic heart failure due to left ventricular systolic dysfunction. Eur J Heart Fail 2007;9(3):243–50.

[11] Chan J, Sanderson J, Chan W, et al. Prevalence of sleep-disordered breathing in diastolic heart failure. Chest 1997;111(6):1488–93.

[12] Vasan RS, Larson MG, Benjamin EJ, et al. Congestive heart failure in subjects with normal versus reduced left ventricular ejection fraction: prevalence and mortality in a population-based cohort. J Am Coll Cardiol 1999;33(7):1948–55.

[13] Chaudhary BA, Ferguson DS, Speir WA Jr. Pulmonary edema as a presenting feature of sleep apnea syndrome. Chest 1982;82(1):122–4.

[14] Hedner J, Ejnell H, Caidahl K. Left ventricular hypertrophy independent of hypertension in patients with obstructive sleep apnoea. J Hypertens 1990;8(10):941–6.

[15] Noda A, Okada T, Yasuma F, et al. Cardiac hypertrophy in obstructive sleep apnea syndrome. Chest 1995;107(6):1538–44.

[16] Alchanatis M, Tourkohoriti G, Kosmas EN, et al. Evidence for left ventricular dysfunction in patients with obstructive sleep apnoea syndrome. Eur Respir J 2002;20(5):1239–45.

[17] Arias MA, Garcia-Rio F, Alonso-Fernandez A, et al. Obstructive sleep apnea syndrome affects left ventricular diastolic function: effects of nasal continuous positive airway pressure in men. Circulation 2005;112(3):375–83.

[18] Kaneko Y, Floras JS, Usui K, et al. Cardiovascular effects of continuous positive airway pressure in patients with heart failure and obstructive sleep apnea. N Engl J Med 2003;348(13):1233–41.

[19] Malone S, Liu PP, Holloway R, et al. Obstructive sleep apnoea in patients with dilated cardiomyopathy: effects of continuous positive airway pressure. Lancet 1991;338(8781):1480–4.

[20] Shivalkar B, Van de HC, Kerremans M, et al. Obstructive sleep apnea syndrome: more insights on structural and functional cardiac alterations, and the effects of treatment with continuous positive airway pressure. J Am Coll Cardiol 2006;47(7):1433–9.

[21] Tolle FA, Judy WV, Yu PL, et al. Reduced stroke volume related to pleural pressure in obstructive sleep apnea. J Appl Physiol 1983;55(6):1718–24.

[22] Parker JD, Brooks D, Kozar LF, et al. Acute and chronic effects of airway obstruction on canine left ventricular performance. Am J Respir Crit Care Med 1999;160(6):1888–96.

[23] Levy PA, Guilleminault C, Fagret D, et al. Changes in left ventricular ejection fraction during REM sleep and exercise in chronic obstructive pulmonary disease and sleep apnoea syndrome. Eur Respir J 1991;4(3):347–52.

[24] Cloward TV, Walker JM, Farney RJ, et al. Left ventricular hypertrophy is a common echocardiographic abnormality in severe obstructive sleep apnea and reverses with nasal continuous positive airway pressure. Chest 2003;124(2):594–601.

[25] Cohn JN, Ferrari R, Sharpe N. Cardiac remodeling–concepts and clinical implications: a consensus paper from an international forum on cardiac remodeling. Behalf of an International Forum on Cardiac Remodeling. J Am Coll Cardiol 2000;35(3):569–82.

[26] Virolainen J, Ventila M, Turto H, et al. Effect of negative intrathoracic pressure on left ventricular pressure dynamics and relaxation. J Appl Physiol 1995;79(2):455–60.

[27] Somers V, Javaheri S. Cardiovascular effects of sleep-related breathing disorders. In: Kryger MH, Roth T, Dement WC, editors. Principles and practices of sleep medicine. 4th edition. Philadelphia: WB Saunders; 2005. p. 1180–91.

[28] Brinker JA, Weiss JL, Lappe DL, et al. Leftward septal displacement during right ventricular loading in man. Circulation 1980;61(3):626–33.

[29] Chen L, Einbinder E, Zhang Q, et al. Oxidative stress and left ventricular function with chronic intermittent hypoxia in rats. Am J Respir Crit Care Med 2005;172(7):915–20.

[30] Nakao K, Ohgushi M, Yoshimura M, et al. Hyperventilation as a specific test for diagnosis of coronary artery spasm. Am J Cardiol 1997; 80(5):545–9.

[31] Arabi Y, Morgan BJ, Goodman B, et al. Daytime blood pressure elevation after nocturnal hypoxia. J Appl Physiol 1999;87(2):689–98.

[32] Somers VK, Mark AL, Zavala DC, et al. Contrasting effects of hypoxia and hypercapnia on ventilation and sympathetic activity in humans. J Appl Physiol 1989;67(5):2101–6.

[33] Narkiewicz K, Montano N, Cogliati C, et al. Altered cardiovascular variability in obstructive sleep apnea. Circulation 1998;98(11):1071–7.

[34] Dyugovskaya L, Lavie P, Lavie L. Increased adhesion molecules expression and production of reactive oxygen species in leukocytes of sleep apnea patients. Am J Respir Crit Care Med 2002; 165(7):934–9.

[35] Schulz R, Mahmoudi S, Hattar K, et al. Enhanced release of superoxide from polymorphonuclear neutrophils in obstructive sleep apnea. Impact of continuous positive airway pressure therapy. Am J Respir Crit Care Med 2000;162(2 Pt 1): 566–70.

[36] Zhang GX, Kimura S, Nishiyama A, et al. Cardiac oxidative stress in acute and chronic isoproterenol-infused rats. Cardiovasc Res 2005;65(1): 230–8.

[37] Aoki M, Nata T, Morishita R, et al. Endothelial apoptosis induced by oxidative stress through activation of NF-kappaB: antiapoptotic effect of antioxidant agents on endothelial cells. Hypertension 2001;38(1):48–55.

[38] Tanaka M, Ito H, Adachi S, et al. Hypoxia induces apoptosis with enhanced expression of Fas antigen messenger RNA in cultured neonatal rat cardiomyocytes. Circ Res 1994;75(3):426–33.

[39] Phelan MW, Faller DV. Hypoxia decreases constitutive nitric oxide synthase transcript and protein in cultured endothelial cells. J Cell Physiol 1996;167(3):469–76.

[40] Ip MS, Lam B, Chan LY, et al. Circulating nitric oxide is suppressed in obstructive sleep apnea and is reversed by nasal continuous positive airway pressure. Am J Respir Crit Care Med 2000; 162(6):2166–71.

[41] Imadojemu VA, Gleeson K, Quraishi SA, et al. Impaired vasodilator responses in obstructive sleep apnea are improved with continuous positive airway pressure therapy. Am J Respir Crit Care Med 2002;165(7):950–3.

[42] Bokinsky G, Miller M, Ault K, et al. Spontaneous platelet activation and aggregation during obstructive sleep apnea and its response to therapy with nasal continuous positive airway pressure. A preliminary investigation. Chest 1995;108(3): 625–30.

[43] Shamsuzzaman AS, Winnicki M, Lanfranchi P, et al. Elevated C-reactive protein in patients with obstructive sleep apnea. Circulation 2002; 105(21):2462–4.

[44] Chen L, Shi Q, Scharf SM. Hemodynamic effects of periodic obstructive apneas in sedated pigs with congestive heart failure. J Appl Physiol 2000;88(3):1051–60.

[45] Kita H, Ohi M, Chin K, et al. The nocturnal secretion of cardiac natriuretic peptides during obstructive sleep apnoea and its response to therapy with nasal continuous positive airway pressure. J Sleep Res 1998;7(3):199–207.

[46] Somers VK, Dyken ME, Mark AL, et al. Sympathetic-nerve activity during sleep in normal subjects. N Engl J Med 1993;328(5):303–7.

[47] Horner RL, Brooks D, Kozar LF, et al. Immediate effects of arousal from sleep on cardiac autonomic outflow in the absence of breathing in dogs. J Appl Physiol 1995;79(1):151–62.

[48] Garpestad E, Katayama H, Parker JA, et al. Stroke volume and cardiac output decrease at termination of obstructive apneas. J Appl Physiol 1992; 73(5):1743–8.

[49] Eichhorn EJ, Bristow MR. Medical therapy can improve the biological properties of the chronically failing heart. A new era in the treatment of heart failure. Circulation 1996;94(9): 2285–96.

[50] Sutton MG, Sharpe N. Left ventricular remodeling after myocardial infarction: pathophysiology and therapy. Circulation 2000;101(25): 2981–8.

[51] Daly PA, Sole MJ. Myocardial catecholamines and the pathophysiology of heart failure. Circulation 1990;82(Suppl 2):I35–43.

[52] Floras JS. Clinical aspects of sympathetic activation and parasympathetic withdrawal in heart failure. J Am Coll Cardiol 1993;22(4 Suppl A): 72A–84A.

[53] Kaye DM, Lambert GW, Lefkovits J, et al. Neurochemical evidence of cardiac sympathetic activation and increased central nervous system norepinephrine turnover in severe congestive heart failure. J Am Coll Cardiol 1994;23(3):570–8.

[54] Verdecchia P, Schillaci G, Guerrieri M, et al. Circadian blood pressure changes and left ventricular hypertrophy in essential hypertension. Circulation 1990;81(2):528–36.

[55] Portaluppi F, Provini F, Cortelli P, et al. Undiagnosed sleep-disordered breathing among male nondippers with essential hypertension. J Hypertens 1997;15(11):1227–33.

[56] Brooks D, Horner RL, Kozar LF, et al. Obstructive sleep apnea as a cause of systemic hypertension. Evidence from a canine model. J Clin Invest 1997;99(1):106–9.

[57] Fletcher EC, Proctor M, Yu J, et al. Pulmonary edema develops after recurrent obstructive apneas. Am J Respir Crit Care Med 1999;160 (5 Pt 1):1688–96.

[58] Tkacova R, Rankin F, Fitzgerald FS, et al. Effects of continuous positive airway pressure on obstructive sleep apnea and left ventricular afterload in patients with heart failure. Circulation 1998;98(21):2269–75.

[59] Sin DD, Fitzgerald F, Parker JD, et al. Relationship of systolic BP to obstructive sleep apnea in patients with heart failure. Chest 2003;123(5): 1536–43.

[60] Bradley TD, Hall MJ, Ando S, et al. Hemodynamic effects of simulated obstructive apneas in humans with and without heart failure. Chest 2001;119(6):1827–35.

[61] Carlson JT, Rangemark C, Hedner JA. Attenuated endothelium-dependent vascular relaxation in patients with sleep apnoea. J Hypertens 1996; 14(5):577–84.

[62] Schulz R, Hummel C, Heinemann S, et al. Serum levels of vascular endothelial growth factor are elevated in patients with obstructive sleep apnea and severe nighttime hypoxia. Am J Respir Crit Care Med 2002;165(1):67–70.

[63] Alchanatis M, Paradellis G, Pini H, et al. Left ventricular function in patients with obstructive sleep apnoea syndrome before and after treatment with nasal continuous positive airway pressure. Respiration 2000;67(4):367–71.

[64] Hanly P, Sasson Z, Zuberi N, et al. Ventricular function in snorers and patients with obstructive sleep apnea. Chest 1992;102(1):100–5.

[65] Laaban JP, Cassuto D, Orvoen-Frija E, et al. Cardiorespiratory consequences of sleep apnoea syndrome in patients with massive obesity. Eur Respir J 1998;11(1):20–7.

[66] Laaban JP, Pascal-Sebaoun S, Bloch E, et al. Left ventricular systolic dysfunction in patients with obstructive sleep apnea syndrome. Chest 2002; 122(4):1133–8.

[67] Alonso-Fernandez A, Garcia-Rio F, Arias MA, et al. Obstructive sleep apnoea-hypoapnoea syndrome reversibly depresses cardiac response to exercise. Eur Heart J 2006;27(2):207–15.

[68] Alonso-Fernandez A, Arias M, Garcia-Rio F. Determining Cardiac Output by Carbon Dioxide Rebreathing in Patients With Sleep Apnea-Hypopnea Syndrome. Arch Bronconeumol 2006; 42(2):92–5.

[69] Fung JW, Li TS, Choy DK, et al. Severe obstructive sleep apnea is associated with left ventricular diastolic dysfunction. Chest 2002;121(2):422–9.

[70] Sidana J, Aronow WS, Ravipati G, et al. Prevalence of moderate or severe left ventricular diastolic dysfunction in obese persons with obstructive sleep apnea. Cardiology 2005;104(2): 107–9.

[71] Kasikcioglu HA, Karasulu L, Durgun E, et al. Aortic elastic properties and left ventricular diastolic dysfunction in patients with obstructive sleep apnea. Heart Vessels 2005;20(6):239–44.

[72] Amin RS, Kimball TR, Kalra M, et al. Left ventricular function in children with sleep-disordered breathing. Am J Cardiol 2005;95(6):801–4.

[73] Bhatia RS, Tu JV, Lee DS, et al. Outcome of heart failure with preserved ejection fraction in a population-based study. N Engl J Med 2006;355(3):260–9.

[74] Shepard JW Jr, Pevernagie DA, Stanson AW, et al. Effects of changes in central venous pressure on upper airway size in patients with obstructive sleep apnea. Am J Respir Crit Care Med 1996; 153(1):250–4.

[75] Arzt M, Young T, Finn L, et al. Sleepiness and sleep in patients with both systolic heart failure and obstructive sleep apnea. Arch Intern Med 2006;166(16):1716–22.

[76] Ross J Jr. Afterload mismatch and preload reserve: a conceptual framework for the analysis of ventricular function. Prog Cardiovasc Dis 1976;18(4):255–64.

[77] Carlson JT, Hedner J, Elam M, et al. Augmented resting sympathetic activity in awake patients with obstructive sleep apnea. Chest 1993; 103(6):1763–8.

[78] Hedner J, Ejnell H, Sellgren J, et al. Is high and fluctuating muscle nerve sympathetic activity in the sleep apnoea syndrome of pathogenetic importance for the development of hypertension? J Hypertens Suppl 1988;6(4):S529–31.

[79] Somers VK, Dyken ME, Clary MP, et al. Sympathetic neural mechanisms in obstructive sleep apnea. J Clin Invest 1995;96(4):1897–904.

[80] Oldenburg O, Lamo B, Faber L, et al. Sleep-disordered breathing in patients with symptomatic heart failure A contemporary study of prevalence in and characteristics of 700 patients. Eur J Heart Fail 2007;9(3):251–7.

[81] Pepperell JC, Ramdassingh-Dow S, Crosthwaite N, et al. Ambulatory blood pressure after therapeutic and subtherapeutic nasal continuous positive airway pressure for obstructive sleep apnoea: a randomised parallel trial. Lancet 2002;359(9302): 204–10.

[82] Engleman HM, Martin SE, Deary IJ, et al. Effect of continuous positive airway pressure treatment on daytime function in sleep apnoea/hypopnoea syndrome. Lancet 1994;343(8897):572–5.

[83] Barbe F, Mayoralas LR, Duran J, et al. Treatment with continuous positive airway pressure is not effective in patients with sleep apnea but no daytime sleepiness: a randomized, controlled trial. Ann Intern Med 2001;134(11):1015–23.

[84] Krieger J, Grucker D, Sforza E, et al. Effects of long-term treatment with nasal continuous positive airway pressure. Chest 1991;100(4):917–21.

[85] Arias MA, Garcia-Rio F, Alonso-Fernandez A, et al. Pulmonary hypertension in obstructive sleep apnoea: effects of continuous positive airway pressure: a randomized, controlled crossover study. Eur Heart J 2006;27(9):1106–13.

[86] Mansfield DR, Gollogly NC, Kaye DM, et al. Controlled trial of continuous positive airway pressure in obstructive sleep apnea and heart failure. Am J Respir Crit Care Med 2004; 169(3):361–6.

[87] Narkiewicz K, Kato M, Phillips BG, et al. Nocturnal continuous positive airway pressure decreases daytime sympathetic traffic in obstructive sleep apnea. Circulation 1999;100(23): 2332–5.

[88] Chin K, Ohi M, Kita H, et al. Effects of NCPAP therapy on fibrinogen levels in obstructive sleep apnea syndrome. Am J Respir Crit Care Med 1996;153(6 Pt 1):1972–6.

[89] Tkacova R, Dajani HR, Rankin F, et al. Continuous positive airway pressure improves nocturnal baroreflex sensitivity of patients with heart failure and obstructive sleep apnea. J Hypertens 2000;18(9):1257–62.

[90] Bradley TD, Holloway RM, McLaughlin PR, et al. Cardiac output response to continuous positive airway pressure in congestive heart failure. Am Rev Respir Dis 1992;145(2 Pt 1):377–82.

[91] Kraiczi H, Hedner J, Peker Y, et al. Comparison of atenolol, amlodipine, enalapril, hydrochlorothiazide, and losartan for antihypertensive treatment in patients with obstructive sleep apnea. Am J Respir Crit Care Med 2000;161(5):1423–8.

[92] Javaheri S. Effects of continuous positive airway pressure on sleep apnea and ventricular irritability in patients with heart failure. Circulation 2000;101:392–7.

SLEEP
MEDICINE
CLINICS

Sleep Med Clin 2 (2007) 575–581

ELSEVIER
SAUNDERS

Obstructive Sleep Apnea and Arrhythmias

Suraj Kapa, MD[a], Shahrokh Javaheri, MD[b],
Virend K. Somers, MD, PhD[c],*

- Mechanisms of arrhythmogenesis
  - *Physiology of normal sleep*
  - *Arrhythmias during sleep*
  - *The diving reflex*
- Bradyarrhythmias
- Atrial fibrillation

- Ventricular ectopy and arrhythmias
- Sudden cardiac death
- Treatment of arrhythmias in sleep apnea
- Summary
- References

Obstructive sleep apnea (OSA) may independently, or in association with other cardiovascular triggers (such as ischemic heart disease or heart failure), predispose patients to the development of arrhythmias [1]. The Sleep Heart Health Study demonstrated that individuals with severe sleep-disordered breathing had two- to four-fold higher odds of developing complex arrhythmias than those without sleep-disordered breathing [2]. These arrhythmias primarily occur during sleep hours and include either brady- or tachyarrhythmias. The mechanisms by which obstructive sleep apnea contributes to arrhythmogenesis may include increased sympathetic nerve activity, reflex increases in vagal tone, hypoxemia, or by decreasing arrhythmia threshold.

Mechanisms of arrhythmogenesis

Disordered cardiac rhythm may occur in sleep apnea patients, even in the absence of conduction system disease [3]. Dysrhythmias may include bradycardia [4], heart block [5,6], atrial fibrillation [7,8], and ventricular ectopy and tachycardia [4]. The pathogenesis of these rhythm changes relates to dysfunction in the normal sleep cycle, hypoxemia, changes in autonomic tone, and lowering of ischemic thresholds, thus raising arrhythmogenic potential. An understanding of the pathogenesis of dysrhythmias in sleep apnea requires an understanding of the normal physiology of sleep, of the normal response to apnea in healthy persons, and of the response to obstructed apneas in OSA patients.

Physiology of normal sleep

Physiologically, sleep consists of nonrapid eye movement and rapid eye movement (REM) components. Each of these stages is associated with characteristic changes in autonomic tone, with non-REM sleep being associated with decreased sympathetic and increased parasympathetic activity—resulting

[a] Division of Internal Medicine, Mayo Clinic College of Medicine, 200 First Street SW, Rochester, MN 55905, USA
[b] Sleepcare Diagnostics, 4780 Socialville-Fosters Road, Mason, OH 45040, USA
[c] Division of Cardiovascular Diseases and Internal Medicine, Mayo Clinic College of Medicine, 200 First Street SW, Rochester, MN 55905, USA
* Corresponding author.
E-mail address: somers.virend@mayo.edu (V.K. Somers).

1556-407X/07/$ – see front matter © 2007 Elsevier Inc. All rights reserved.   doi:10.1016/j.jsmc.2007.07.009
sleep.theclinics.com

in decreases in heart rate and blood pressure—and phasic REM sleep being associated with heightened peripheral sympathetic drive, surges in blood pressure, and irregular heart rate, with bursts of cardiac vagotonia. As a result of these variations in autonomic tone throughout the sleep cycle, there are effects on normal cardiac electrophysiology. Increased parasympathetic activity during sleep may result in marked sinus arrhythmias, type I or II atrioventricular block, and sinus pauses in otherwise healthy people [9,10]. Disordered sleep may further aggravate any predisposition to sleep-associated rhythm disturbances.

Arrhythmias during sleep

Arrhythmias during sleep may be either supraventricular or ventricular in origin. Ventricular arrhythmias, similar to cardiovascular events, demonstrate a diurnal variation, peaking in incidence in the early morning [11,12]. This tendency may be related in part to the decreased ischemic threshold in the early morning, which occurs temporally with diurnal variation in sympathetic activity, endothelial function, and coagulability. Ischemia alone can act as a stimulus for the development of arrhythmias and thus may play an important role in early morning arrhythmogenesis [13].

Arrhythmogenesis may also be related to autonomic surges. For example, an abrupt increase in vagal or sympathetic activity during REM sleep may predispose to the development of arrhythmias [13]. Another example is vagal-induced atrial fibrillation, which may occur during sleep when there is a profound parasympathetic predominance [14]. These variations in resting autonomic tone may act in the absence of an abnormal cardiac substrate to cause rhythm disturbances during early morning wakefulness. These disturbances may be more pronounced, or the arrhythmic threshold may be decreased, in patients with an underlying substrate, such as coronary artery disease, myocardial ischemia or infarction, or heart failure, or with OSA, which elicits hypoxemia and marked alterations in vagal and sympathetic drive.

The diving reflex

Sleep apnea is associated with prolonged episodes of breathing cessation with associated hypoxia. The response to prolonged apneic episodes in diving mammals and in human beings during sustained submersion under water may mimic the physiology seen in patients with sleep apnea. The usual physiologic response to hypoxia is an increase in ventilation. However, prolonged hypoxia, secondary to an absence of breathing, is unique in that oxygen stores are not repleted, so the body responds by maintaining oxygen delivery to the vital organs—the brain and the heart—while decreasing oxygen delivery to the rest of the body via sympathetic vasoconstriction. This state of elevated sympathetic tone does not affect blood flow to the brain, because the cerebral vasculature is under autoregulatory control, nor to the heart. An increase in cardiac parasympathetic tone results in bradycardia and a resultant decrease in myocardial oxygen demand. These physiologic changes allow for increased brain and heart survival under conditions of anoxia associated with prolonged apnea.

Bradyarrhythmias

Bradyarrhythmias are the most frequent arrhythmias seen in OSA. These include both sinus bradycardia and atrioventricular block, varying from sinus arrest (Fig. 1) to complete heart block and ventricular asystole [15]. Pathophysiologically, the major contributing factor to bradyarrhythmias in sleep apnea is a chemoreceptor mediated increase in vagal tone caused by apnea and hypoxemia [16–18]. In terms of normal physiology, this increase in vagal tone is consistent with that seen in the diving reflex, when prolonged apnea causes an increase in sympathetic tone to the peripheral blood vessels and increased vagal drive to the heart.

Bradyarrhythmias typically occur in the absence of any known conduction system disease. In addition, there is an association between disease severity and the occurrence of bradycardia [4,19], with bradycardia more likely to appear when sleep apnea is most severe (during REM sleep) [19,20]. A causal relationship is suggested in these patients by a greater likelihood for dysrhythmia during and immediately after apneic episodes [21].

Bradyarrhythmias in the sleep apnea population are often asymptomatic because episodes of rhythm disturbance only occur at night [22]. Furthermore, these bradyarrhythmias can be prevented by treating the underlying sleep apnea [4,19,22–24]. This has been suggested in trials using either tracheostomy or continuous positive airway pressure (CPAP) for treatment of sleep apnea, further suggesting a causal relationship between sleep apnea and bradyarrhythmia. In fact, CPAP therapy has been shown to be curative in patients with asymptomatic nocturnal bradyarrhythmia referred for pacemaker therapy [25]. As demonstrated in studies of atrial overdrive pacing, it has been further proposed that treatment of underlying rhythm disturbances may also play a role in attenuating sleep apnea episodes [26]. However, subsequent studies showed that pacemaker

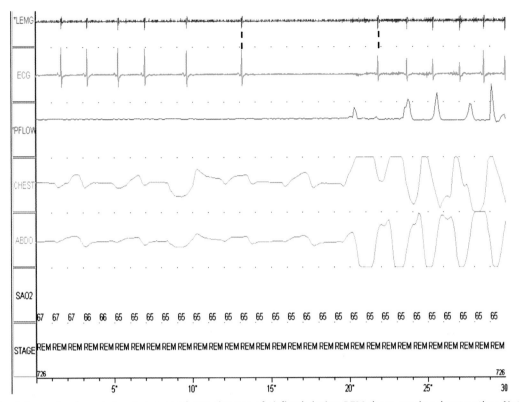

Fig. 1. Example of an obstructive apnea (note absence of airflow) during REM sleep, causing desaturation. Note progressive decrease in heart rate followed by sinus arrest. ECG changes are also observed on leg electromyogram tracing.

placement is of little benefit in treating obstructive sleep apnea [27,28].

Thus, patients who present with asymptomatic bradyarrhythmias occurring during sleep should be screened for the presence of sleep apnea. Screening for treatment of sleep apnea could potentially avoid a more invasive procedure, such as pacemaker implantation. Nevertheless, if bradyarrhythmias do not resolve with treatment of OSA, appropriate treatment of any conduction failure should be initiated.

Atrial fibrillation

There is a strong association between atrial fibrillation and OSA [29], which may be explained by functional and structural effects of sleep apnea on the heart. These include hypoxemia associated with prolonged apneic episodes, intrathoracic pressure oscillations causing increased cardiac wall stress [30,31], autonomic imbalances during apnea [32], and diastolic dysfunction [33]. Long-term atrial remodeling in patients with sleep apnea may also contribute to a predisposition to developing atrial fibrillation. The coprevalence of atrial fibrillation and sleep apnea may also be more pronounced in patients with an underlying cardiac abnormality, such as heart failure [34]. Furthermore, sleep-disordered breathing diagnosed preoperatively may predict atrial fibrillation after coronary bypass surgery [7].

The relationship between atrial fibrillation and OSA appears to be independent of gender, hypertension, heart failure, or body mass index. Obesity and the magnitude of nocturnal oxygen desaturation in patients with sleep apnea are also independent risk factors for atrial fibrillation in patients less than 65 years of age [35]. The presence of untreated sleep apnea in patients with atrial fibrillation doubles the likelihood of recurrence within 12 months of cardioversion, when compared with those receiving treatment [36]. However, some data suggest that atrial fibrillation recurrence may be similar in patients at high risk for sleep apnea and in those at low risk for sleep apnea, as seen on long-term pacemaker recordings of atrial fibrillation recurrence [37].

Ventricular ectopy and arrhythmias

The relationship between ventricular arrhythmias and sleep apnea remains to be fully elucidated.

Some studies have shown that premature ventricular contractions more frequently occur with pronounced oxygen desaturation [38]. The frequency of ventricular ectopy in this patient population may be related to the aforementioned increased likelihood of bradyarrhythmias. Episodes of ventricular asystole associated with significantly reduced heart rate may predispose these patients to developing ventricular escape beats, partly accounting for the noted increase in ventricular ectopy. In patients with heart failure, treatment of coexisting sleep apnea by CPAP reduces the frequency of ventricular premature beats, suggesting a correlative role between the two [39,40].

Ventricular tachycardia has also been reported in sleep apnea [4,41], though the prevalence and severity and the clinical significance of these arrhythmias in sleep apnea remains unclear. The association between sleep apnea and ventricular arrhythmias is stronger in the presence of other underlying cardiac disease, such as heart failure [42,43] or after coronary artery bypass surgery, suggesting that the relationship between ventricular arrhythmias and sleep apnea is one of decreased threshold and exacerbation of underlying cardiac disease.

This association is further supported by the relationship between ischemia and sleep apnea. Patients with sleep apnea showed a greater incidence of cardiac arrhythmias during an acute myocardial infarction, though these patients had the same clinical course during hospitalization and similar mortality rates to non-sleep apnea patients [44]. In contrast, another study in patients with mild to moderate sleep-disordered breathing and coronary artery disease, suggested an increased frequency of premature ventricular contractions and higher heart rates, but no difference in frequency of serious ventricular arrhythmias [45]. A possible relationship between sleep apnea and ventricular arrhythmia, however, is supported by a reported decrease in arrhythmias in this patient population after CPAP therapy [40].

Sudden cardiac death

Nocturnal arrhythmias in patients with sleep apnea may potentially be related to the higher nighttime prevalence of sudden cardiac death in this population (Fig. 2) [46]. In the general population, sudden cardiac death, myocardial infarction and ventricular arrhythmias show a day-night variation, with a preponderance in the early morning hours, between 6 AM and noon. In patients with sleep apnea, the peak in sudden death occurs during sleeping hours, between midnight and 6 AM, while in the general population the nadir in sudden death from cardiac causes occurs during this time period [47]. The severity of sleep apnea correlates with the risk of nocturnal sudden death [46]. While OSA changes the timing of sudden death, whether OSA increases the risk of sudden death remains unknown. Nevertheless, the increased arrhythmogenic potential in sleep apnea suggests that recognition and treatment may possibly be important in improving morbidity and mortality in this population.

Treatment of arrhythmias in sleep apnea

Treatment of sleep apnea may attenuate the arrhythmogenic potential of apneic episodes in sleep apnea patients [48]. This is true for bradyarrhythmias and perhaps also atrial fibrillation [49] and ventricular arrhythmias. Recognition of the role of treating sleep apnea, as a means of avoiding

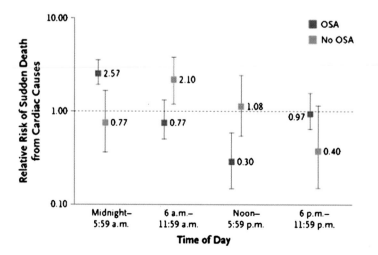

Fig. 2. Relative risk of sudden death from cardiac causes. (*From* Gami AS, Howard DE, Olson EJ, et al. Day-night pattern of sudden death in obstructive sleep apnea. N Engl J Med 2005;352:1211; with permission. Copyright ©2005, Massachusetts Medical Society.)

the need for pacemakers in this patient population with otherwise asymptomatic nocturnal bradyarrhythmias, is important [50].

The benefits of atrial overdrive pacing in reducing the apnea-hypopnea index in patients with sleep apnea are limited. Pacing may play a role in relieving asymptomatic nocturnal bradycardia and atrioventricular block. Furthermore, one recent study suggested that in pacemaker patients with sleep-related issues, using a sleep rate function on the pacemaker could improve both the quality and the quantity of sleep [51]. However, there is evidence that temporary atrial pacing does not improve the respiratory manifestations of obstructive sleep apnea [27,28]. CPAP therapy has also been shown to be significantly better in treating OSA than overdrive pacing [52].

Summary

There is a relationship between arrhythmias and sleep apnea, most notably during sleep. The most common rhythm disturbance is nocturnal bradyarrhythmias that occur in association with apneic episodes. However, because of long-term autonomic, functional, and structural cardiac changes, in addition to decreased ischemic threshold, patients with sleep apnea may potentially be at higher risk for developing atrial fibrillation and ventricular arrhythmias. These complications of untreated sleep apnea may be implicated in nocturnal sudden cardiac death. However, there are not yet any definitive data identifying OSA as a cause of either atrial fibrillation or ventricular arrhythmias. Nevertheless, it is possible that treatment of sleep apnea, using standard modalities such as CPAP or tracheostomy, may reduce the incidence and the recurrence of arrhythmias in this population.

References

[1] Somers V, Javaheri S. Cardiovascular effects of sleep-related breathing disorders. In: Kryger MH, Roth T, Dement WC, editors. Principles and practices of sleep medicine. 4th edition. Philadelphia: WB Saunders; 2005. p. 1180–91.

[2] Mehra R, Benjamin EJ, Shahar E, et al. Association of nocturnal arrhythmias with sleep-disordered breathing: the Sleep Heart Health Study. Am J Respir Crit Care Med 2006;173:910–6.

[3] Hoffstein V, Mateika S. Cardiac arrhythmias, snoring, and sleep apnea. Chest 1994;106: 466–71.

[4] Guilleminault C, Connolly SJ, Winkle RA. Cardiac arrhythmia and conduction disturbances during sleep in 400 patients with sleep apnea syndrome. Am J Cardiol 1983;52:490–4.

[5] Becker HF, Koehler U, Stammnitz A, et al. Heart block in patients with sleep apnoea. Thorax 1998;53:S29–32.

[6] Rama PR, Sharma SC. Sleep apnea and complete heart block. Clin Cardiol 1994;17:675–7.

[7] Mooe T, Gullsby S, Rabben T, et al. Sleep-disordered breathing: a novel predictor of atrial fibrillation after coronary artery bypass surgery. Coron Artery Dis 1996;7:475–8.

[8] Coccagna G, Capucci A, Bauleo S, et al. Paroxysmal atrial fibrillation in sleep. Sleep 1997;20: 396–8.

[9] Nevins DB. First- and second-degree A-V heart block with rapid eye movement sleep. Ann Intern Med 1972;76:981–3.

[10] Guilleminault C, Pool P, Motta J, et al. Sinus arrest during REM sleep in young adults. N Engl J Med 1984;311:1006–10.

[11] Raeder EA, Hohnloser SH, Graboys TB, et al. Spontaneous variability and circadian distribution of ectopic activity in patients with malignant ventricular arrhythmias. J Am Coll Cardiol 1988; 12:656–61.

[12] Englund A, Behrens S, Wegscheider K, et al. Circadian variation of malignant ventricular arrhythmias in patients with ischemic and nonischemic heart disease after cardioverter defibrillator implantation. European 7219 Jewel Investigators. J Am Coll Cardiol 1999;34: 1560–8.

[13] Wolk R, Gami AS, Garcia-Touchard A, et al. Sleep and cardiovascular disease. Curr Probl Cardiol 2005;30:625–62.

[14] Singh J, Mela T, Ruskin J. Images in cardiovascular medicine. Sleep (vagal)-induced atrial fibrillation. Circulation 2004;110:e32–3.

[15] Simantirakis EN, Schiza SI, Marketou ME, et al. Severe bradyarrhythmias in patients with sleep apnoea: the effect of continuous positive airway pressure treatment: a long-term evaluation using an insertable loop recorder. Eur Heart J 2004;25: 1070–6.

[16] De Burgh Daly M, Angell-James JE, Elsner R. Role of carotid-body chemoreceptors and their reflex interactions in bradycardia and cardiac arrest. Lancet 1979;1:764–7.

[17] Somers VK, Dyken ME, Mark AL, et al. Parasympathetic hyperresponsiveness and bradyarrhythmias during apnoea in hypertension. Clin Auton Res 1992;2:171–6.

[18] Zwillich C, Devlin T, White D, et al. Bradycardia during sleep apnea: characteristics and mechanism. J Clin Invest 1982;69:1286–92.

[19] Becker H, Brandenberg U, Peter JH, et al. Reversal of sinus arrest and atrioventricular condiction block in patients with sleep apnea during nasal continuous positive airway pressure. Am J Respir Crit Care Med 1995;151:215–8.

[20] Koehler U, Becker HF, Grimm W, et al. Relations among hypoxemia, sleep stage, and

bradyarrhythmia during obstructive sleep apnea. Am Heart J 2000;139:142–8.

[21] Szaboova E, Donic V, Albertova D, et al. [Nocturnal cardiac dysrhythmias associated with obstructive sleep apnea]. Sb Lek 2002;103:79–83 [in Slovak].

[22] Grimm W, Koehler U, Fus E, et al. Outcome of patients with sleep apnea-associated severe bradyarrhythmias after continuous positive airway pressure therapy. Am J Cardiol 2000;86:688–92.

[23] Koehler U, Fus E, Grimm W, et al. Heart block in patients with obstructive sleep apnea: pathogenetic factors and effects of treatment. Eur Respir J 1998;11:434–9.

[24] Grimm W, Hoffman J, Menz V, et al. Electrophysiologic evaluation of sinus node function and atrioventricular conduction in patients with prolonged ventricular asystole during obstructive sleep apnea. Am J Cardiol 1996;77:1310–4.

[25] Stegman SS, Burroughs JM, Henthorn RW. Asymptomatic bradyarrhythmias as a marker for sleep apnea: appropriate recognition and treatment may reduce the need for pacemaker therapy. Pacing Clin Electrophysiol 1996;19:899–904.

[26] Garrigue S, Bordier P, Jais P, et al. Benefit of atrial pacing in sleep apnea syndrome. N Engl J Med 2002;346:404–12.

[27] Krahn AD, Yee R, Erickson MK, et al. Physiologic pacing in patients with obstructive sleep apnea: a prospective, randomized crossover trial. J Am Coll Cardiol 2006;47:379–83.

[28] Pepin JL, Defaye P, Garrigue S, et al. Overdrive atrial pacing does not improve obstructive sleep apnoea syndrome. Eur Respir J 2005;25:343–7.

[29] Gami AS, Pressman G, Caples SM, et al. Association of atrial fibrillation and obstructive sleep apnea. Circulation 2004;110:364–7.

[30] Schafer H, Hasper E, Ewig S, et al. Pulmonary haemodynamics in obstructive sleep apnoea: time course and associated factors. Eur Respir J 1998;12:679–84.

[31] Tkacova R, Rankin F, Fitzgerald FS, et al. Effects of continuous positive airway pressure on obstructive sleep apnea and left ventricular afterload in patients with heart failure. Circulation 1998;98:2269–75.

[32] Roche F, Xuong AN, Court-Fortune I, et al. Relationship among the severity of sleep apnea syndrome, cardiac arrhythmias, and autonomic imbalance. Pacing Clin Electrophysiol 2003;26:669–77.

[33] Fung JW, Li TS, Choy DK, et al. Severe obstructive sleep apnea is associated with left ventricular diastolic dysfunction. Chest 2002;121:422–9.

[34] Javaheri S, Parker TJ, Liming JD, et al. Sleep apnea in 81 ambulatory male patients with stable heart failure. Types and their prevalences, consequences, and presentations. Circulation 1998;97:2154–9.

[35] Gami AS, Hodge DO, Herges RM, et al. Obstructive sleep apnea, obesity, and the risk of incident atrial fibrillation. J Am Coll Cardiol 2007;49:565–71.

[36] Kanagala R, Murali NS, Friedman PA, et al. Obstructive sleep apnea and the recurrence of atrial fibrillation. Circulation 2003;107:2589–94.

[37] Padeletti L, Gensini GF, Pieragnoli P, et al. The risk profile for obstructive sleep apnea does not affect the recurrence of atrial fibrillation. Pacing Clin Electrophysiol 2006;29:727–32.

[38] Shepard JW, Garrison MW, Grither DA, Dolan GF. Relationship of ventricular ectopy to oxyhemoglobin desaturation in patients with obstructive sleep apnea. Chest 1985;88:335–40.

[39] Ryan CM, Usui K, Floras JS, et al. Effect of continuous positive airway pressure on ventricular ectopy in heart failure patients with obstructive sleep apnoea. Thorax 2005;60:781–5.

[40] Javaheri S. Effects of continuous positive airway pressure on sleep apnea and ventricular irritability in patients with heart failure. Circulation 2000;101:392–7.

[41] Koehler U, Glaremin T, Cassel W, et al. [Nocturnal ventricular arrhythmia in patients with sleep apnea and suspected coronary artery disease]. Med Klin (Munich) 1993;88:684–90 [in German].

[42] Fichter J, Bauer D, Arampatzis S, et al. Sleep-related breathing disorders are associated with ventricular arrhythmias in patients with an implantable cardioverter-defibrillator. Chest 2002;122:558–61.

[43] Javaheri S, Corbett WS. Association of low PaCO$_2$ with central sleep apnea and ventricular arrhythmias in ambulatory patients with stable heart failure. Ann Intern Med 1998;128:204–7.

[44] Marin JM, Carrizo SJ, Kogan I. Obstructive sleep apnea and acute myocardial infarction: clinical implications of the association. Sleep 1998;21:809–15.

[45] Mooe T, Franklin KA, Wiklund U, et al. Cardiac rhythm in patients with sleep-disordered breathing and coronary artery disease. Scand Cardiovasc J 2000;34:272–6.

[46] Gami AS, Howard DE, Olson EJ, et al. Day-night pattern of sudden death in obstructive sleep apnea. N Engl J Med 2005;352:1206–14.

[47] Cohen MC, Rohtla KM, Lavery CE, et al. Meta-analysis of the morning excess of acute myocardial infarction and sudden cardiac death. Am J Cardiol 1997;79:1512–6.

[48] Harbison J, O'Reilly P, McNicholas WT. Cardiac rhythm disturbances in the obstructive sleep apnea syndrome: effects of nasal continuous positive airway pressure therapy. Chest 2000;118:591–5.

[49] Gami AS, Friedman PA, Chung MK, et al. Therapy insight: interactions between atrial

fibrillation and obstructive sleep apnea. Nat Clin Pract Cardiovasc Med 2005;2:145–9.

[50] Grimm W, Becker HF. Obesity, sleep apnea syndrome, and rhythmogenic risk. Herz 2006;31:213–8.

[51] Greco OT, Bittencourt LR, Vargas RN, et al. Sleep parameters in patients using pacemakers with sleep rate function on. Pacing Clin Electrophysiol 2006;29:135–41.

[52] Unterberg C, Luthje L, Szych J, et al. Atrial overdrive pacing compared to CPAP in patients with obstructive sleep apnea syndrome. Eur Heart J 2005;26:2568–75.

ELSEVIER
SAUNDERS

SLEEP
MEDICINE
CLINICS

Sleep Med Clin 2 (2007) 583–591

Sleep Apnea and Stroke: A Risk Factor or an Association?

Henry Yaggi, MD, MPH[a,b], Vahid Mohsenin, MD[b],*

- Sleep-disordered breathing and stroke
- Sleep apnea, cognitive impairment, and white matter disease
- Pathophysiologic mechanisms in sleep apnea leading to stroke
  Cerebral hemodynamics in normal sleep and sleep apnea
- *Cardiac arrhythmia*
- *Abnormal coagulation markers*
- *Atherosclerosis*
- Therapy for sleep apnea and impact on cerebrovascular risk
- Summary
- References

It is estimated that around 59 million people will die in 2007. One disease, stroke, will kill 10% of these, and leave millions of others disabled. Stroke ranks as the second leading cause of death worldwide, and it is the leading cause of disability among adults [1]. Understanding underlying pathophysiology, promoting preventative behaviors, and developing novel therapeutic approaches for stroke is of crucial importance. Stroke is a heterogeneous disorder that encompasses various subtypes (Box 1). Ischemic stroke is the most common form of stroke. Within this type is a self-limited form of stroke known as "transient ischemic attack," which lasts less than 24 hours. With the more widespread use of modern brain imaging, many patients with symptoms lasting less than 24 hours are found to have an infarction. Despite years of research, alteplase, a recombinant tissue plasminogen activator, is still the only approved treatment of acute stroke and is only effective in limiting stroke insult if given within 3 hours of stroke onset. Many patients with stroke are either passed this narrow

intervention window or simply do not have access to alteplase. Primary prevention of stroke should be the primary goal for the reduction in morbidity and mortality from this devastating disease. There are several modifiable risk factors for stroke that include hypertension, cardiac disease, atrial fibrillation, diabetes mellitus, dyslipidemia, smoking, alcohol abuse, sedentary life style, and hypercoagulable state [2]. Understanding the link between obstructive sleep apnea syndrome (OSAS) and stroke may represent one such novel approach. Recent studies indicate that OSAS may serve as an independent risk factor for the development of stroke [3,4], and therapy for OSAS may help to reduce cardiovascular and cerebrovascular risk [5]. OSAS is defined as apnea-hypopnea index of greater than or equal to 5 per hour sleep and associated symptoms of sleepiness, cognitive dysfunction, and cardiovascular complications.

This article explores the relationship between OSAS and stroke by critically reviewing the current literature. First, epidemiologic studies are analyzed

[a] Section of Pulmonary and Critical Care Medicine, Clinical Epidemiology Research Center, VA Connecticut Healthcare System, 950 Campbell Avenue, West Haven, CT 06516, USA
[b] Section of Pulmonary and Critical Medicine, Yale University School of Medicine, 40 Temple Street, Suite 3C, New Haven, CT 06510, USA
* Corresponding author.
E-mail address: vahid.mohsenin@yale.edu (V. Mohsenin).

1556-407X/07/$ – see front matter © 2007 Elsevier Inc. All rights reserved.
sleep.theclinics.com

doi:10.1016/j.jsmc.2007.07.004

> **Box 1:   Classification and distribution of cerebrovascular disease**
>
> Ischemic stroke 86%
>
> - Transient ischemic attack 20%
> - Thrombotic 48%
> - Embolic 18%
>
> Hemorrhagic stroke 14%
>
> - Intracerebral 8%
> - Subarachnoid 6%

with respect to issues regarding the strength of the association, and the consistency of the association using different study designs and different populations. Next, the biologic plausibility of the relationship is explored by reviewing studies that examine the pathophysiology of sleep apnea and stroke. Subsequently, studies exploring the therapeutic impact of OSAS on stroke and cardiovascular risk are reviewed. Finally, public health implications are discussed.

Sleep-disordered breathing and stroke

OSAS is characterized by repeated episodes of upper airway obstruction and is often associated with snoring, arterial oxygen desaturation, acute surges in pulmonary and systemic arterial blood pressure, and sleep disruption. Early epidemiologic studies showed an association between snoring and stroke. These studies also demonstrated the strength of this association to be similar to traditional risk factors for stroke, such as hypertension, smoking, atrial fibrillation, and hypercholesterolemia. Furthermore, even when adjusted for confounding risk factors, such as obesity, hypertension, age, and gender, there remained an independent association between snoring and stroke [6–13]. More robust evidence came from several large prospective studies, which seem to corroborate the earlier case-control and cross-sectional studies. In an early cohort study exclusively of Finnish men, there was a twofold increase in the relative risk for the combined outcome of stroke and ischemic heart disease in habitual snorers compared with nonsnorers [7]. A smaller but still significant positive association (relative risk, 1.33) between regular snoring and the combined cardiovascular outcome of stroke and ischemic heart disease was seen in women in the Nurses Health Study [13].

Although snoring is a common occurrence in OSAS, it is not the same as obstructive apnea. A number of cross-sectional and case-control studies have used overnight polysomnography to define OSAS more precisely, to sort out whether it is the

minority of patients with OSAS who account for the apparent increased risk of snoring with stroke (Table 1). These studies have focused on OSAS both as a consequence of stroke and as a risk factor for the development of stroke [14–19].

An early study of 10 patients recovering from hemispheric stroke revealed a high prevalence (80%) of obstructive sleep apneas compared with age and body mass index–matched controls with similar frequency of hypertension and smoking without stroke [14]. The mean respiratory disturbance index (sum of apneas and hypopnea per hour sleep) for the stroke group was 52 events per hour compared with 3 in the control group. In a similar study, OSAS was diagnosed in 19% of the controls and 71% of the stroke patients [16]. The mean lowest arterial oxygen saturation level was 91% in the control group and 85% in the stroke group, and the mean respiratory disturbance index was 4 events per hour for controls and 26 events per hour for stroke patients. The 4-year mortality for patients with stroke was 21%, and all patients with stroke who died (of various causes) had OSAS. Stronger epidemiologic evidence demonstrating the association between sleep-disordered breathing and cerebrovascular disease comes from the initial results of Sleep Heart Health Study [19]. This community-based study explored the association between sleep-disordered breathing and prevalent self-reported cardiovascular disease (myocardial infarction, angina, coronary revascularization procedures, heart failure, or stroke) in a large cohort of 6424 individuals who underwent unattended overnight polysomnography at home. This study showed a positive association (odds ratio 1.42; 95% confidence interval, 1.13–1.78) between patients with an apnea-hypopnea index greater than 11 and prevalent cardiovascular events. The designs of these initial studies were predominantly case-control or cross-sectional and subject to recall bias. An additional limitation was the inability to establish the temporal relationship between stroke and OSAS because snoring and OSAS can be a consequence of stroke. In the absence of a sleep study demonstrating OSAS preceding the stroke, it is difficult to be certain that OSAS is a consequence of the stroke. The direction of the arrow of causation can ultimately only be definitively determined by analysis of incident cerebrovascular disease events. More recently, several large prospective observational cohort studies have demonstrated that OSAS increases the risk for stroke [3], stroke and all-cause-mortality [4], and fatal and nonfatal cardiovascular events [5] independent of known risk factors. Furthermore, a significant trend was noted showing increasing severity of OSAS was associated with higher risk of stroke or death. Those patients in

Table 1: Selected studies of sleep apnea and stroke using polysomnography

Study	Study Design	Number of Patients/ Controls	Mean RDI	Study Population	Confounding Assessment	Prevalence Sleep Apnea in Stroke (%)
Mohsenin and Valor [14]	Case-control	10/10	52	Predominantly hemispheric stroke in a rehabilitation unit	Age, BMI, hypertension, smoking	80% with RDI ≥20
Good et al [15]	Descriptive	47 (19 underwent PSG)	NA	Rehabilitation patients recently hospitalized for stroke	NA	32% had ≥10 desaturation events per hour based on computerized overnight oximetry
Dyken et al [16]	Case-control	24/19	26	Recently hospitalized for stroke	Age, gender	71% with RDI ≥10
Bassetti and Aldrich [17]	Case-control	128/25 (80 underwent PSG)	28	Inpatients with stroke and TIA	Age, BMI, diabetes, severity of stroke	63% with RDI ≥10
Para et al [18]	Descriptive	161	21	Inpatients with stroke and TIA	NA	71% with RDI ≥10 [a](acute phase) 61% with RDI ≥10 (stable phase)
Shahar et al [19]	Cross-sectional (Sleep Heart Health Study)	6/424	NA (see text)	Assembled from several ongoing population-based studies of CVD in the United States	Age, race, gender, smoking, diabetes, hypertension, BMI, cholesterol	NA (see text) [a]RR of stroke comparing lowest quartile with highest quartile = 1.58 with 95% CI (1.02–2.46)

Abbreviations: BMI, body mass index; CI, confidence interval; CVD, cerebrovascular disease; NA, not applicable; PSG, polysomnography; RDI, respiratory disturbance index, which is the number of apneas plus hypopneas per hour of sleep; RR, relative risk; TIA, transient ischemic attack.
[a] Acute phase after admission and stable phase indicates >3 months later.

the highest severity quartile of the cohort (apnea-hypopnea index >36) had a greater than threefold increased risk for the development of stroke or death. Taken together, these data point toward OSAS as an independent cerebrovascular risk factor.

Sleep apnea, cognitive impairment, and white matter disease

Epidemiologic studies, primarily in middle-aged adults, have shown associations between OSAS and deficits in cognitive functioning, particularly attention and concentration [20,21]. These deficits may, in part, be mediated through the excessive daytime sleepiness associated with OSAS. Even after adequate therapy for OSAS, some cognitive deficits,

such as impairment in executive functioning and manual dexterity, can persist [22,23]. The residual deficits may, in part, be related to repeated exposure to hypoxia and cerebral hemodynamic perturbation causing structural changes in the brain. Elderly patients with white matter disease, as demonstrated on CT, are more likely to have severe OSAS compared with those without white matter disease [24]. In a younger population of patients with OSAS, however, there was no difference in the prevalence of white matter disease compared with controls without OSAS. This difference between the younger and the older population with white matter disease may be explained by the duration of exposure to OSAS and its hemodynamic consequences.

the activation of proinflammatory mediators, including adhesion molecules and cytokines. It has been demonstrated that OSAS increases circulating levels of adhesion molecules, such as intercellular adhesion molecule-1, VCAM-1 (vascular cell adhesion molecule), interleukin-8, and MCP-1 (monocyte chemoattractant protein-1) [74–76].

Some recent work has examined inflammatory biomarkers of cardiovascular risk in patients with OSAS. One study compared levels of C-reactive protein (a nonspecific marker of inflammation and risk factor for atherosclerosis) and interleukin-6 (a proinflammatory cytokine that is also implicated in the pathogenesis of atherosclerosis) between patients with OSAS and obesity-matched controls. Both levels were significantly higher in patients with OSAS and then decreased with CPAP treatment [77]. In addition to supporting the association of OSAS and cardiovascular risk, this study also demonstrates the potential for serologic markers of cardiovascular risk in patients with OSAS.

Although these studies have provided significant insight to the potential mechanisms by which OSAS may lead to stroke, their actual role in the pathogenesis of cerebrovascular disease in the setting of OSAS remains to be established. Interventional studies are needed to link these biomarkers in the prevention of stroke.

Therapy for sleep apnea and impact on cerebrovascular risk

Prospective observational cohort studies have demonstrated that CPAP therapy reduces the risk of fatal and nonfatal cardiovascular outcomes [5], confers a protective effect against death from cardiovascular disease [78], and reduces mortality in patients with severe OSAS [79].

At the time of this writing, there are no prospective studies examining the effect of treatment of OSAS on primary prevention of stroke, but there is accumulating indirect evidence for stroke risk reduction with the treatment of OSAS. In a double-blind, placebo-controlled, randomized trial comparing therapeutic with sham CPAP, therapeutic airway pressurization was associated with a 3 to 7 mm Hg reduction in mean 24-hour blood pressure [30]. In extrapolating from pharmacologic antihypertensive trials, this blood pressure reduction, in itself, is expected to result in a 20% stroke risk reduction [80]. Much like the impact of β-blockade on the risk of myocardial infarction, however, the beneficial impact of CPAP therapy on the risk of stroke is expected to extend beyond just that associated with blood pressure reduction. Indeed, CPAP therapy stabilizes oxygenation; reduces

sympathetic activity and catecholamine levels [28]; improves left ventricular function [81]; decreases platelet aggregation [68], plasma fibrinogen levels [60], and inflammatory markers of atherosclerosis [77]; and reduces risk of atrial fibrillation [51].

Summary

Recent prospective cohort studies have demonstrated that OSAS is associated with a twofold to threefold increased risk of developing stroke independent of known cerebrovascular risk factors. Plausible mechanisms underlying this risk of stroke are multifactorial and include hypertension, changes in cerebral hemodynamics, paradoxical embolism, cardiac arrhythmias, hypercoagulability, and progression of atherosclerosis. Long-term therapy with CPAP may help to reduce risk of fatal and nonfatal cardiovascular and possibly cerebrovascular outcomes.

References

[1] Murray C, Lopex A. Mortality by cause for eight regions of the world: Global Burden of Disease Study. Lancet 1997;349:1269–76.

[2] Sacco RL, Adams R, Albers G, et al. Guidelines for prevention of stroke in patients with ischemic stroke or transient ischemic attack: a statement for healthcare professionals from the American Heart Association/American Stroke Association Council on Stroke: co-sponsored by the Council on Cardiovascular Radiology and Intervention: the American Academy of Neurology affirms the value of this guideline. Circulation 2006; 113(10):e409–49.

[3] Arzt M, Young T, Finn L, et al. Association of sleep-disordered breathing and the occurrence of stroke. Am J Respir Crit Care Med 2005;172: 1447–51.

[4] Yaggi H, Concato J, Kernan W, et al. Obstructive sleep apnea as a risk factor for stroke and death. N Engl J Med 2005;353:2034–41.

[5] Marin JM, Carrizo SJ, Vicente E, et al. Long-term cardiovascular outcomes in men with obstructive sleep apnoea-hypopnoea with or without treatment with continuous positive airway pressure: an observational study. Lancet 2005;365(9464): 1046–53.

[6] Partinen M, Palomaki H. Snoring and cerebral infarction. Lancet 1985;2:1325–6.

[7] Koskenvuo M, Kaprio J, Telakivi T, et al. Snoring as a risk factor for ischaemic heart disease and stroke in men. Br Med J (Clin Res Ed) 1987; 294:16–9.

[8] Spriggs D, French J, Murdy J, et al. Snoring increases the risk of stroke and adversely affects prognosis. Q J Med 1992;83:555–62.

[9] Palomaki H. Snoring and the risk of ischemic brain infarction. Stroke 1991;22:1021–5.

[10] Smirne S, Palazzi S, Zucconi M, et al. Habitual snoring as a risk factor for acute vascular disease. Eur Respir J 1993;6:1357–61.

[11] Jennum P, Schultz-Larsen K, Davidsen M, et al. Snoring and risk of stroke and ischaemic heart disease in a 70 year old population: a 6-year follow-up study. Int J Epidemiol 1994;23(6):1159–64.

[12] Neau J, Meurice J, Paquereau J, et al. Habitual snoring as a risk factor for brain infarction. Acta Neurol Scand 1995;92:63–8.

[13] Hu F, Willet W, Manson J, et al. Snoring and the risk of cardiovascular disease in women. J Am Coll Cardiol 2000;35:308–13.

[14] Mohsenin V, Valor R. Sleep apnea in patients with hemispheric stroke. Arch Phys Med Rehabil 1995;76:71–6.

[15] Good D, Henkle J, Gelber D, et al. Sleep-disordered breathing and poor functional outcome after stroke. Stroke 1996;27:252–9.

[16] Dyken M, Somers V, Yamada T, et al. Investigating the relationship between stroke and obstructive sleep apnea. Stroke 1996;27:401–7.

[17] Bassetti C, Aldrich M. Sleep apnea in acute cerebrovascular diseases: final report on 128 patients. Sleep 1999;22:217–23.

[18] Parra O, Arboix A, Bechich S, et al. Time course of sleep-related breathing disorders in first-ever stroke or transient ischemic attack. Am J Respir Crit Care Med 2000;161:375–80.

[19] Shahar E, Whitney C, Redline S, et al. Sleep-disordered breathing and cardiovascular disease: cross-sectional results of the Sleep Heart Health Study. Am J Respir Crit Care Med 2001;163:19–25.

[20] Kim H, Young T, Mathews C, et al. Sleep-disordered breathing and neuropsychological deficits. Am J Respir Crit Care Med 1997;156:1813–9.

[21] Redline S, Strauss ME, Adams N, et al. Neuropsychological function in mild sleep-disordered breathing. Sleep 1997;20:160–7.

[22] Sforza E, Krieger J. Daytime sleepiness after long-term continuous positive airway pressure (CPAP) treatment in obstructive sleep apnea syndrome. J Neurol Sci 1992;110(1–2):21–6.

[23] Bedard MA, Montplaisir J, Malo J, et al. Persistent neuropsychological deficits and vigilance impairment in sleep apnea syndrome after treatment with continuous positive airways pressure (CPAP). J Clin Exp Neuropsychol 1993;15(2):330–41.

[24] Harbison J, Gibson GJ, Birchall D, et al. White matter disease and sleep-disordered breathing after acute stroke. Neurology 2003;61(7):959–63.

[25] Leung R, Bradley T. Sleep apnea and cardiovascular disease. Am J Respir Crit Care Med 2001;164:2147–65.

[26] O'Donnell C, King E, Schwartz A, et al. Relationship between blood pressure and airway obstruction during sleep in the dog. J Appl Physiol 1994;(77):1819–28.

[27] Peppard P, Young T, Palta M, et al. Prospective study of the association between sleep-disordered breathing and hypertension. N Engl J Med 2000;342:1378–84.

[28] Faccenda J, Mackay T, Boon N, et al. Randomized placebo-controlled trial of continuous positive airway pressure on blood pressure in the sleep apnea-hypopnea syndrome. Am J Respir Crit Care Med 2001;163:344–8.

[29] Becker H, Jerrentrup A, Ploch T, et al. Effect of nasal continuous positive airway pressure treatment on blood pressure in patients with obstructive sleep apnea. Circulation 2003;107:68–73.

[30] Pepperell J, Ramdassingh-Dow S, Crosthwaite N, et al. Ambulatory blood pressure after therapeutic and subtherapeutic nasal continuous positive airway pressure for obstructive sleep apnoea: a randomised parallel trial. Lancet 2002;359:204–10.

[31] Somers V, Dyken M, Clary M, et al. Sympathetic neural mechanisms in obstructive sleep apnea. J Clin Invest 1995;96:1897–904.

[32] Fletcher E, Orolinova N, Bader M. Blood pressure response to chronic episodic hypoxia: the renin-angiotensin system. J Appl Physiol 2002;92:627–33.

[33] Verdecchia P, Schillaci G, Guerrieri M. Circadian blood pressure changes and left ventricular hypertrophy. Circulation 1990;81:528–36.

[34] O'Brien E, Sheridan J, O'Malley K. Dippers and non-dippers. Lancet 1988;2(8607):397.

[35] Logan A, Tkacova R, Perlikowski S, et al. Refractory hypertension and sleep apnea: effect of CPAP on blood pressure and baroreflex. Eur Respir J 2003;21:241–7.

[36] Madsen P, Schmidt J, Holm S, et al. Cerebral oxygen metabolism and cerebral blood flow in man during light sleep (stage 2). Brain Res 1991;557:217–20.

[37] Diomedi M, Placidi F, Cupini L, et al. Cerebral hemodynamic changes in sleep apnea syndrome and effect of continuous positive airway pressure treatment. Neurology 1998;51:1051–6.

[38] Droste D, Berger W, Schuler E, et al. Middle cerebral artery blood flow velocity in healthy persons during wakefulness and sleep: a transcranial Doppler study. Sleep 1993;16:603–9.

[39] Fischer A, Chaudry B, Taormina M, et al. Intracranial hemodynamics in sleep apnea. Chest 1992;102:1402–6.

[40] Hoshi Y, Mizukami S, Tamura M. Dynamic features of hemodynamic and metabolic changes in human brain during all-night sleep as revealed by near-infrared spectroscopy. Brain Res 1994;652:257–62.

[41] Lenzi P, Zoccoli G, Walker A, et al. Cerebral blood flow regulation in REM sleep: a model for flow metabolism coupling. Arch Ital Biol 1999;137:165–79.

[42] Sakai F, Meyer J, Karacan I, et al. Normal human sleep: regional cerebral hemodynamics. Ann Neurol 1980;7:471–8.

[43] Klingelhofer J, Hajak G, Matzander G, et al. Dynamics of cerebral blood flow velocities

during normal human sleep. Clin Neurol Neurosurg 1995;97:142–8.

[44] Siebler M, Nachtmann A. Cerebral hemodynamics in obstructive sleep apnea. Chest 1993;103:1118–9.

[45] Balfors E, Franklin K. Impairment in cerebral perfusion during obstructive sleep apneas. Am J Respir Crit Care Med 1994;150:1587–91.

[46] Netzer N, Werner P, Jochums I, et al. Blood flow of the middle cerebral artery with sleep-disordered breathing: correlation with obstructive hypopneas. Stroke 1998;29:87–93.

[47] Franklin K. Cerebral haemodynamics in obstructive sleep apnoea and Cheyne-Stokes respiration. Sleep Med Rev 2002;6:429–41.

[48] Fichter J, Bauer D, Arampatzis S, et al. Sleep-related breathing disorders are associated with ventricular arrhythmias in patients with an implantable cardioverter defibrillator. Chest 2002;122:558–61.

[49] Zwillich C, Devlin T, White D, et al. Bradycardia during sleep apnea: characteristics and mechanism. J Clin Invest 1982;69:1286–92.

[50] Javaheri S, Parker T, Liming J, et al. Sleep apnea in 81 ambulatory male patients with stable heart failure: types and their prevalences, consequences, and presentations. Circulation 1998;97:2154–9.

[51] Kanagala R, Murali N, Friedman P, et al. Obstructive sleep apnea and the recurrence of atrial fibrillation. Circulation 2003;107:2589–94.

[52] Di Minno G, Mancini M. Measuring plasma fibrinogen to predict stroke and myocardial infarction. Arteriosclerosis 1990;10:1–7.

[53] Kannel W, Wolf P, Castelli W, et al. Fibrinogen and risk of cardiovascular disease: the Framingham Study. JAMA 1987;258:1183–6.

[54] Meade T, North W, Chakrabarti R, et al. Haemostatic function and cardiovascular death: early results of a prospective study. Lancet 1980;1:1050–4.

[55] Resch K, Ernst E, Matrai A, et al. Fibrinogen and viscosity as risk factors for subsequent cardiovascular events in stroke survivors. Ann Intern Med 1992;117:371–5.

[56] Toss H, Lindhaul B, Siegbahn A, et al. Prognostic influence of increased fibrinogen and C-reactive protein levels in unstable coronary artery disease. Frisc Study Group. Fragmin during instability in coronary artery disease. Circulation 1997;96:4204–10.

[57] Wilhelmsen L, Svardsudd K, Kristoffer K, et al. Fibrinogen as a risk factor stroke and myocardial infarction. N Engl J Med 1984;311:501–5.

[58] Eber B, Schumacher M. Fibrinogen: its role in the hemostatic in atherosclerosis. Semin Thromb Hemost 1993;19:104–7.

[59] Smith E, Keen G, Grant A, et al. Fate of fibrinogen in human arterial intima. Arteriosclerosis 1990;10:263–75.

[60] Chin K, Ohi M, Kita H, et al. Effects of NCPAP therapy on fibrinogen levels in obstructive sleep apnea syndrome. Am J Respir Crit Care Med 1996;153:1972–6.

[61] Steiner S, Jax T, Evers S, et al. Altered blood rheology in obstructive sleep apnea as a mediator of cardiovascular risk. Cardiology 2005;104:92–6.

[62] Wessendorf T, Thilmann A, Wang Y, et al. Fibrinogen levels and obstructive sleep apnea in ischemic stroke. Am J of Respir Crit Care Med 2000;162:2039–42.

[63] Elwood P, Renaud S, Sharp D, et al. Ischemic heart disease and platelet aggregation. The Caerphilly Collaborative Heart Disease Study. Circulation 1991;83:38–44.

[64] Fitzgerald D, Roy L, Catella F, et al. Platelet activation in unstable coronary disease. N Engl J Med 1986;315:983–9.

[65] Thaulow E, Erikssen J, Sandvik L. Blood platelet count and function are related to total and cardiovascular death in apparently healthy men. Circulation 1991;84:613–7.

[66] Trip M, Cats V, Van Capelle F. Platelet hyperreactivity and prognosis in survivors of myocardial function. N Engl J Med 1990;322:1549–54.

[67] Toffler G, Brezinski D, Shafer A, et al. Concurrent morning increase in platelet aggregability and the risk of myocardial infarction and sudden cardiac death. N Engl J Med 1987;316:1514–8.

[68] Bokinsky G, Miller M, Ault K, et al. Spontaneous platelet activation and aggregation during obstructive sleep apnea and its response to therapy with nasal continuous positive airway pressure: a preliminary investigation. Chest 1995;108:625–30.

[69] Dimsdale J, Coy T, Ziegler M, et al. The effect of sleep apnea on plasma and urinary catecholamines. Sleep 1995;18:377–81.

[70] Fletcher E, Miller J, Schaaf J. Urinary catecholamines before and after tracheostomy in patients with obstructive sleep apnea and hypertension. Sleep 1987;10:35–44.

[71] Wedzicha J, Syndercombe-Court D, Tan K. Increased platelet aggregate formation in patients with chronic airflow obstruction and hypoxemia. Thorax 1991;46:504–7.

[72] Hayashi M, Fujimoto K, Urushibata K, et al. Nocturnal oxygen desaturation correlates with the severity of coronary atherosclerosis in coronary artery disease. Chest 2003;124:936–41.

[73] Lavie L. Obstructive sleep apnoea syndrome: an oxidative stress disorder. Sleep Med Rev 2003;7:35–51.

[74] Dyugovskaya L, Lavie P, Lavie L. Increased adhesion molecule expression and production of reactive oxygen species in leukocytes of sleep apnea patients. Am J Respir Crit Care Med 2002;165:934–9.

[75] El-Solh A, Mador M, Sikka P, et al. Adhesion molecules in patients with coronary artery disease and moderate-to-severe obstructive sleep apnea. Chest 2002;121:1541–7.

[76] Ohga E, Nagase T, Tomita T, et al. Increased levels of circulating I-CAM-1, VCAM-1, and L-selectin in obstructive sleep apnea syndrome. J Appl Physiol 1999;87:10–4.

[77] Yokoe T, Minoguchi K, Matsuo H, et al. Elevated levels of C-reactive protein and interleukin-6 in patients with obstructive sleep apnea syndrome are decreased by nasal continuous positive airway pressure. Circulation 2003;107:1129–34.

[78] Doherty LS, Kiely JL, Swan V, et al. Long-term effects of nasal continuous positive airway pressure therapy on cardiovascular outcomes in sleep apnea syndrome. Chest 2005;127(6): 2076–84.

[79] Marti S, Sampol G, Munoz X, et al. Mortality in severe sleep apnoea/hypopnoea syndrome patients: impact of treatment. Eur Respir J 2002; 20:1511–8.

[80] Collins R, Peto R, MacMahon S, et al. Blood pressure, stroke, and coronary heart disease. Part 2, Short-term reductions in blood pressure: overview of randomised drug trials in their epidemiological context. Lancet 1990;335(8693): 827–38.

[81] Kaneko Y, Floras J, Usui K, et al. Cardiovascular effects of continuous positive airway pressure in patients with heart failure and obstructive sleep apnea. N Engl J Med 2003;348:1233–41.

SLEEP
MEDICINE
CLINICS

Sleep Med Clin 2 (2007) 593–601

ELSEVIER
SAUNDERS

Mortality in Obstructive Sleep Apnea

Jose M. Marin, MD[a,b,*], Santiago J. Carrizo, MD[a,b]

- Mortality as an outcome
  - *Markers of disease severity in obstructive sleep apnea*
  - *Cohort versus randomized controlled trials*
- Obesity and mortality
- Mortality studies in obstructive sleep apnea before 1995
- Mortality studies in obstructive sleep apnea after 1995

- The Zaragoza sleep cohort study
- Effect of continuous positive airway pressure on mortality in obstructive sleep apnea
- Summary
- References

Obstructive sleep apnea (OSA) is a frequent disease that affects 4% of middle-age men and 2% of middle-age women [1,2]. OSA is characterized by recurrent collapse of the pharyngeal airway during sleep. In those episodes, respiratory effort is present and arterial oxygen saturation decreases, terminated by an arousal from sleep. The two main clinical consequences of OSA are daytime sleepiness and cardiovascular sequelae, which are responsible for the potential increased morbidity and mortality associated with this condition (Fig. 1). Increased traffic accidents in untreated OSA patients compared with non-OSA patients have been demonstrated [3,4], but the cardiovascular consequences of OSA are still a subject of debate [5,6]. This article examines the growing evidence that links OSA with cardiovascular outcomes and specifically with an excess of mortality.

Mortality as an outcome

The term "outcome" is designed to evaluate the consequences of the disease as experienced by the patient, death being the main outcome of any medical entity. In OSA, outcomes include daytime sleepiness; snoring; morning hangover; poor health-related quality of life; increased health resource use; cardiovascular outcomes (systemic hypertension, myocardial infarction, stroke, congestive heart disease); and death (Box 1). Some clinical outcomes, such as drowsiness or snoring, are easily measured within routine practice and in the setting of a clinical trial and are very sensitive to medical intervention [7,8]. Others, such as cardiovascular outcomes or death, are subjected to comorbid conditions that make it more difficult to establish the specific role of OSA. As a consequence,

[a] Respiratory Service, Hospital Universitario Miguel Servet, 1-3, Isabel la Católica Avenue, 50009-Zaragoza, Spain
[b] University of Zaragoza, Zaragoza, Spain
* Corresponding author. Respiratory Service, Hospital Universitario Miguel Servet, 1-3, Isabel la Católica Avenue, 50009-Zaragoza, Spain.
E-mail address: jmmarint@unizar.es (J.M. Marin).

1556-407X/07/$ – see front matter © 2007 Elsevier Inc. All rights reserved.
sleep.theclinics.com

doi:10.1016/j.jsmc.2007.07.001

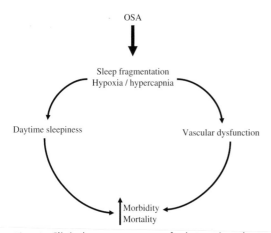

Fig. 1. Clinical consequences of obstructive sleep apnea.

in OSA, studies designed to evaluate the effects of treatment directly on cardiovascular and mortality outcomes are impracticable and unethical, because these clinical outcomes may need to run for a long time in otherwise symptomatic patients for whom an effective treatment is available [9]. Death is the strongest outcome in clinical trials. Some studies done in the cardiology field with antihypertensive drugs have shown that the active drug produced a modest reduction in blood pressure numbers and no modification in left ventricular ejection fraction [10]. Because the active drug also showed an increase in survival, however, these medications are included in the treatment guidelines of chronic heart failure.

Markers of disease severity in obstructive sleep apnea

A "marker" is a measurement known to be associated with a clinical outcome. In OSA, the best widely accepted marker of disease severity is the apnea-hypopnea index (AHI), which is the number of apneas and hypopneas per hour of sleep. The

Box 1: Hierarchy of clinical outcomes in OSA

Death
Cardiovascular

   Nonfatal myocardial infarction
   Nonfatal stroke or transient ischemic attack
   Heart failure
   Pulmonary hypertension
   Cardiac arrhythmias
   Systemic hypertension

Traffic accidents
Health quality of life
Daytime sleepiness

AHI is used not only to define the OSA syndrome (AHI >5 plus daytime sleepiness) but also serves to stratify OSA severity: mild OSA (AHI between 5 and 15); moderate OSA (AHI between 16 and 30); and severe OSA (AHI >30) [11]. Some have argued that this classification is arbitrary, because there are little data evaluating the relationship between the AHI and daytime symptom severity. Nevertheless, recent studies proved helpful in OSA severity stratification by AHI as a marker for cardiovascular morbidity and mortality in long-term cohort studies [12–14]. Oxygen desaturation, sleep disruption, and total sleep time are important pathologic processes that go together with apnea episodes. It is possible that these factors act as markers of disease severity and outcomes in OSA, but there are even less data on the literature addressing the issue. Until a gold standard marker is widely accepted, AHI could be considered the best surrogate of OSA severity as a sleep-disordered breathing.

Cohort versus randomized controlled trials

Evidence for an association of a marker and an outcome comes from different kinds of studies that can be grouped (Fig. 2). Randomized controlled trials are the most robust tools because they have fewer biases and have proved to have the best inference. Cross-sectional studies are often flawed by confounding variables, which are unknown before the study is designed, so they provide weaker and more biased inference. Most epidemiologists consider cohort observational studies as suggestive of an association between specific markers and outcomes, but with no definitive proof of that relationship. The main criticism is that in the observational studies the effects of an intervention (eg, nasal continuous positive airway pressure [CPAP] in OSA) may be caused by an unrecognized confounding factor rather than the effect of treatment. Well-conducted randomized controlled trials have the clear advantage over observational studies in that they control for both known and unknown or unmeasured confounding factors, such as life course socioeconomic position and doctor selection practices. They are not always feasible, however, and because of the expense and ethical concerns of randomized trials, it is important that observational studies be

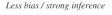
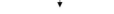

- Randomized controlled trials   *Less bias / strong inference*

- Cohort Studies

- Case Control

- Case Series

- Cross-sectional studies   *More bias / weaker inference*

Fig. 2. Levels of evidence in clinical studies.

used effectively to direct investigators to the interventions most appropriately assessed by trials.

In OSA there are no long-term randomized controlled trials assessing the natural history of the disease and the therapy impact on robust fatal and nonfatal cardiovascular outcomes. These studies are only feasible in asymptomatic patients because the symptomatic should receive an effective treatment, such as nasal CPAP. Nevertheless, several reviews have suggested that well-planned observational studies provide information that closely resembles that provided by randomized trials [15,16].

Obesity and mortality

Most patients with OSA are overweight or obese. Obesity is associated with reduced chest wall compliance, decreased lung volumes, and increased upper airway resistance [17]. Adiposity of the neck also promotes the collapse of upper airway during sleep [18]. All of these factors contribute to increase the severity of the nocturnal respiratory events, and there is a linear relationship between body weight and the frequency of respiratory events during sleep [19]. Some authors have argued that, because obesity per se carries an increase in cardiovascular morbidity and mortality, it is likely that weight (more specifically upper body obesity) and not the AHI value is responsible for increases in such outcomes [20,21].

Recently, Adams and colleagues [22] published the results of a 10-year follow-up of a very large cohort of men and women in the United States recruited from the general population. They found an increased risk of death with excess body weight. The risk of death increases by 20% to 40% among overweight persons (body mass index [BMI] of 25–29.9 kg/m^2) and by two to at least three times among obese persons (BMI >30 kg/m^2). The results were adjusted for confounding variables, including level of education, race, alcohol consumption, and physical activity. Because OSA symptoms were not recorded and no sleep studies were done, the authors cannot rule out the possibility that sleep apnea accounted for the relationship between adiposity and the risk of death. Obesity is listed as a major modifiable cardiovascular risk factor [22]. Two thirds of patients who have had a myocardial infarction have a BMI greater than 25 [23]. A recent report of a systematic review and meta-analysis of cohort studies examining the association between bodyweight and mortality have provided some conflicting results [24]. Overweight was associated with a better survival and fewer cardiovascular events than normal BMI. Obesity was associated with an increased total mortality only in patients with

a history of coronary artery bypass graft, and severe obesity was associated with the highest cardiovascular mortality but not with increased total mortality. This study confirms the deleterious effect of obesity (BMI >30 kg/m^2), but in some ways it contradicts the study by Adams and colleagues [22]. In the American study the follow-up was 10 years; follow-up here was limited to 3.8 years, which is insufficient to detect the full effect of being overweight on long-term outcomes because the full effect of obesity on cardiovascular mortality may begin after 15 years or more [25].

Obesity and OSA share several pathophysiologic pathways by which both entities increase the risk for developing vascular diseases. They reduce insulin sensitivity enhancing free fatty acid turnover, induce a hypercoagulable state, and promote systemic inflammation, all of which contribute to the development and progression of atherosclerosis [26]. Obesity and OSA are also favorable conditions for developing major cardiovascular risk factors, such as diabetes, dyslipidemia, and hypertension [27,28]. Interestingly, obesity researchers have largely ignored the possibility that results attributed to obesity might be caused by OSA. It is conceivable that OSA is an important part of the mechanism by which obesity leads to cardiovascular disease. If so, this is of fundamental significance because it opens an alternative strategy to address the growing epidemic of obesity.

Besides decreasing lung function, obesity increases cardiovascular risk, making it hard to assess the independent role of OSA on cardiovascular morbidity and mortality. The interrelationships between obesity and OSA are complex and possibly bidirectional, so obesity is a pivotal confounder that needs to be considered very carefully when designing clinical trials.

Mortality studies in obstructive sleep apnea before 1995

In 1997, Wright and colleagues [29] reported a systemic review of all studies published between 1966 and 1995 on the association between OSA and mortality. They argued that at that time there was a paucity of robust evidence for such a relationship. The paper led to a very positive outcome, because it stimulated new approaches and studies. Until 1995 only six articles with mortality as an outcome were published (Table 1). Two were retrospective and the results were not adjusted for BMI and had small samples [30,31]. The other four were prospective and three of them only included elderly population [32–35]. All six studies had many methodologic limitations because they failed adequately to take into account important confounding risk factors

Table 1: **Mortality studies in OSA published before 1996**

Author	Design	Total sample	Mean age	Mean AHI	Mean follow-up	Results
He et al [30]	Retrospective	385	52	35	NA	AI >20 has a RR of 1.5 versus AI <20
Gonzalez-Rothi et al [31]	Retrospective	126	46	39	3 y	RR 1.35 versus control (not significant)
Bliwise et al [32]	Prospective	298	69	NA	Up 12 y	RR of 2.7 for RDI >10 (not significant)
Ancoli-Israel et al [33]	Prospective	233	83	19	3.3 y	Significant association of AHI and death in women but not in men
Mant et al [34]	Prospective	163	83	NA	4 y	No relationship between RDI and survival
Lavie et al [35]	Prospective	1620	48	NA	12 y	OR of 1.012 for AI >10

Abbreviations: AHI, apnea-hypopnea index; AI, apnea index; OR, odds ratio; RDI, respiratory disturbance index; RR, risk ratio.

for cardiovascular diseases, such as obesity, smoking, dyslipemia, or hypertension. Overall, the results of those studies showed inconsistent results with limited evidence to link OSA with an excess of mortality.

Mortality studies in obstructive sleep apnea after 1995

To overcome the limitations of the uncontrolled studies discussed previously, we need well controlled and long-term longitudinal studies. Since the Wright paper was published, at least five longitudinal studies have confirmed increased cardiovascular mortality in OSA patients (Table 2) [12,13,36–38]. Two studies from Sweden compared the mortality of patients with verified coronary

artery disease (CAD) with and without OSA [36,37]. Both used Cox proportional hazards model to identify predictors of end points. In the study by Peker and colleagues [36], after a mean follow-up of 5 years of 62 patients with CAD, the respiratory disturbance index (RDI) remained an independent predictor of cardiovascular mortality (1.13; 95% confidence interval [CI], 1.05–1.21; $P < .001$). In a more powered study (408 patients with CAD), Mooe and colleagues [37] demonstrated that an oxygen desaturation index of greater than 5 predicted a 70% relative increase in the composite end point of death, cerebrovascular events, and myocardial infarction. Similar results were seen in those with an AHI of greater than 10 events per hour. Recently, however, a 10-year survival report did not confirm that OSA worsened the prognosis of patients with

Table 2: **Mortality studies in OSA published after 1996**

Author	Design	Total sample	Mean age	Mean AHI	Mean follow-up	Death results
Peker et al [36]	Prospective	62	68	16	5 y	RR of 1.13 for RDI >10 (significant)
Mooe et al [37]	Prospective	408	60	NA	5 y	RR of 1.60 for ODI >5 (significant)
Lavie et al [38]	Prospective	13,850	48	NA	4.5 y	HR of 2.2 for RDI >30 (significant)
Yaggi et al [13]	Prospective	1022	61	35	3.4 y	HR of 3.3 for AHI >36 (significant)
Marin et al [12]	Prospective	1651	50	32	10 y	OR of 2.87 for AHI >30 (significant)

Abbreviations: AHI, apnea-hypopnea index; AI, apnea index; HR, hazard ratio; OR, odds ratio; RDI, respiratory disturbance index; RR, risk ratio.

CAD [39]. The problem with the latter study is the small number of patients included (N = 50) and the failure to match OSA versus non-OSA groups for age, BMI, and hypertension. It seems that untreated OSA worsens the prognosis of patients with CAD, but the issue is not resolved and more powered studies need to be done in this field.

In OSA patients without pre-existing cardiovascular or cerebrovascular diseases, Yaggi and colleagues [13] reported an increased risk for death or stroke and a dose-effect relationship between OSA severity and risk. This study enrolled 1022 patients; 697 had an AHI greater than 5 and 325 had an AHI less than 5 and were considered the control group. After adjustment for age, gender, race, BMI, smoking and alcohol status, and the presence or absence of major cardiovascular risk, such as diabetes, hyperlipidemia, or hypertension, patients with OSA had an increased risk for the composite primary end point of stroke and death (hazard ratio (HR), 1.97; 95% CI, 1.12–3.48; P = .01). Interesting, in trend analysis, as the severity of AHI increases at baseline, there was an increase risk of the development of the composite end point (P = .005). Patients with severe OSA (AHI >36) had an HR of 3.30 in the composite outcome compared with the control group. This study showed that OSA is a risk for developing first time stroke but it was not apparent if the increase of death rate was caused by vascular causes because all-cause of death was included in the composite outcome. Unfortunately, use of nasal CPAP was not evaluated and the short duration of follow-up (3 years) and the small number of observed events did not allow the specific assessment of the effects of therapy.

All-cause mortality was also evaluated in a recent report from Israel. Lavie and colleagues [38] collected mortality information among a very large cohort of 14,589 men referred to the sleep clinics with suspected sleep apnea. After a median follow-up of 4.6 years, Cox proportional analysis revealed that both BMI and RDI were associated with mortality. The age and the BMI-adjusted hazard ratio for men with a RDI greater than 30 was 2.13 (95% CI, 1.36–2.34) compared with the reference group of patients with a RDI less than 10. In a second and very interesting analysis, the authors compared the relative mortality rates of OSA patients with the general male population in Israel. They found that the increase in all-cause mortality rates among moderate-to-severe RDI categories (RDI >30) was only significantly higher in men aged less than 50 years compared with their counterparts in the general population. The value of this study is the large numbers of patients included and the inclusion of age and BMI as confounders. Unfortunately, no other potential risk of mortality, clinical status at

diagnosis, or therapy was controlled. One important finding in this study is the confirmation of the effect of OSA on mortality in the young and middle aged. Previous less powered studies also have consistently reported that OSA is associated with increased risk of mortality among patients aged less than 50 years with the excessive risk declining after age 50 years [29,33,40]. It seems that the increased risk of mortality reported in OSA was found mainly in younger people and that, as stated by Lavie and colleagues [38], the diagnosis and treatment of sleep apnea should be done at the youngest possible age.

The Zaragoza sleep cohort study

Since the sleep clinic was setup in 1992 in the Hospital Miguel Servet, a tertiary teaching hospital serving a community of up 600,000 people, all patients assessed at baseline are studied under a predetermined protocol. Clinical data are recorded at each outpatient visit using the same standardized questionnaire [41]. Smoking and alcohol consumption status are recorded. The initial evaluation also includes routine blood tests and 12-lead electrocardiography. Blood pressure is measured and hypertension is defined as a systolic blood pressure at rest greater than or equal to 140 mm Hg, a diastolic blood pressure at rest greater than or equal to 90 mm Hg, or treatment with antihypertensive medication [42]. Medical records from hospital and family practitioners are obtained and cardiovascular risk factors are recorded. The diagnosis of diabetes mellitus and other prevalent chronic diseases is established according to the clinical history and use of specific medications, as revealed by the patient or chart review. A full polysomnographic study is obtained in all participants at entry. In keeping with national guidelines, nasal CPAP is recommended to all patients with an AHI greater than or equal to 30 [43]. If the AHI was between 5 and 30, CPAP was equally recommended whenever the patient complained of severe daytime sleepiness that interfered with daily activities or if there was coexistent polycythemia or cardiac failure.

In 2005, the authors reported the long-term cardiovascular outcomes in men with OSA referred to the sleep unit between January 1, 1992, and December 31, 1994 [12]. During the recruitment period 1465 patients had polysomnography and treatment with CPAP was recommended to 667 patients. Patients not treated with nasal CPAP received conservative maneuvers: weight loss; alcohol-sedative avoidance; smoking cessation; avoidance of sleep deprivation; and, if appropriate, sleep position restriction. Patients attended the clinic yearly. During these visits, compliance with CPAP therapy was assessed by the timer built into each CPAP device. A mean daily use of more than 4 hours per day was considered necessary to maintain the CPAP prescription. During the last semester of the year 2003, all patients were contacted by telephone or letter and invited to visit the clinic for examination and to update medical information. There was also the opportunity to evaluate outcomes of healthy male subjects recruited from the Zaragoza Sleep Apnoea Prevalence Study database, a population-based study performed during 1991 and 1992 [41]. In that study, participants completed a general health and a specific sleep questionnaire, and had a polysomnographic study. For the purpose of the current investigation, men who denied excessive daytime somnolence and who did not snore ever as reported by a close relative were selected. Of 277 potential candidates, 268 subjects had an AHI less than 5 and were followed-up.

After a mean of 10.1 years, 264 healthy men, 377 simple snorers, 403 with untreated mild-moderate OSA (AHI <30), 235 with untreated severe OSA (AHI >30), and 372 with OSA treated with CPAP were included in the analysis. Patients with untreated severe OSA had a higher incidence rate of fatal events (1.06 events per 100 person-years) than untreated patients with mild-moderate OSA (0.55 events, <0.02); simple snorers (0.34 events, $P < .0005$); patients treated with nasal CPAP (0.35 events, $P < .005$); and healthy subjects (0.3 events, $P < .005$). Multivariate analysis adjusted for potential confounders showed that untreated severe OSA increased significantly the risk of fatal cardiovascular events (odds ratio 2.87; 95% CI, 1.17–7.51) compared with healthy subjects (Table 3). This was not the case in untreated patients with mild-moderate OSA, simple snorers, or patientstreated with nasal CPAP. It was concluded from this large, long-term, prospective, controlled study that in untreated male patients with severe OSA, the risk of fatal cardiovascular events is increased, there is a dose-effect relationship between the severity of OSA and cardiovascular risk, and simple snoring is not a significant cardiovascular risk factor (Fig. 3). When these results are combined with the previously mentioned revised results, one sees a picture (Fig. 4), in which the risk of death among patients with severe OSA can be considered around 3 times compared with the general population or those of patients with just mild OSA.

Effect of continuous positive airway pressure on mortality in obstructive sleep apnea

Nasal CPAP can effectively treat OSA during sleep [7,8]. Acceptance of CPAP therapy remains a problem in patients without excessive daytime somnolence, however, and in this particular group of nonsleepy patients this device has no benefits [44]. Studies to date regarding the impact of CPAP in OSA used short-term outcomes (<6 months). Few longitudinal studies have assessed death as an outcome until recently. It possible that nasal CPAP decreases the total mortality in OSA patients because it reduces car accidents [45], but no data are definitely available in the literature.

The first study on long-term survival of patients with OSA treated with CPAP was reported by He and colleagues [29]. In their series, none of the patients treated with tracheostomy or nasal CPAP died after a minimum of 5 years. The opposite was found

Table 3: Fully adjusted odds ratio for cardiovascular death associated to clinical variables and diagnosis status, according to the logistic-regression analysis

	OR (95% CI)	P value
Age (y)	1.09 (1.04–1.12)	0.001
Diagnostic group		
Snoring	1.03 (0.31–1.84)	0.88
Mild-moderate OSA	1.15 (0.34–2.69)	0.71
Severe OSA	2.87 (1.17–7.51)	0.025
CPAP	1.05 (0.39–2.21)	0.74
Presence of CV disease	2.54 (1.31–4.99)	0.005

Abbreviations: CPAP, continuous positive airway pressure; CV, cardiovascular; OSA, obstructive sleep apnea.
Data from Marin JM, Carrizo SJ, Vicente E, et al. Long-term cardiovascular outcomes in men with obstructive sleep apnoea-hypopnoea with or without treatment with continuous positive airway pressure: an observational study. Lancet 2005;365:1046–53.

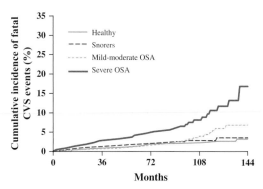

Fig. 3. Cumulative percentage of individuals with fatal cardiovascular events in non-treated with nasal CPAP groups. (*Adapted from* Marin JM, Carrizo SJ, Vicente E, et al. Long-term cardiovascular outcomes in men with obstructive sleep apnoea-hypopnoea with or without treatment with continuous positive airway pressure: an observational study. Lancet 2005;365:1046–53; with permission.)

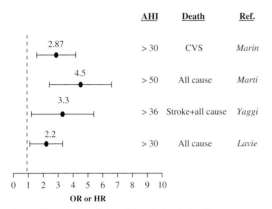

	AHI	Death	Ref.

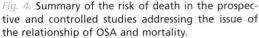

Fig. 4. Summary of the risk of death in the prospective and controlled studies addressing the issue of the relationship of OSA and mortality.

by another noncontrolled study comparing the effect of CPAP with uvulopalatopharyngoplasty; no decrease in survival was found with either therapy compared with no treatment [46]. Both studies lack methodologic precision. More recently, a study from Spain determined survival rates and causes of death in a large group of OSA patients who had been treated with CPAP for a long period of time. This study also analyzed CPAP compliance [47]. They found that mortality rates at 5 years in OSA patients who did not receive CPAP therapy were higher compared with those treated with CPAP (3.4% versus 14.5%; $P < .0001$). Also from Spain, Marti and colleagues [40] reported the long-term survival of a historical large cohort of OSA patients who had been followed-up for up to 14 years. Patients with severe OSA who accepted CPAP and were compliant with the therapy had a reduction of 40% in all-cause mortality compared with those subjects who refused the therapy. The excess cardiovascular fatal events occurred in patients aged less than 50 years who refused CPAP treatment, a finding that supports the high mortality of younger people with untreated OSA. Doherty and colleagues [48] from Ireland also performed a long-term follow-up study of 168 patients with OSA who began CPAP therapy for at least 5 years previously. Incidence of hypertension, ischemic heart disease, and other cardiovascular disorders during follow-up was not significantly different in treated and untreated patients, irrespective of acceptance or refusal of CPAP treatment. Only untreated patients showed excess cardiovascular mortality during follow-up, however, compared with those who accept CPAP (14.8% versus 1.9%).

The authors' sleep cohort study also supports the benefit of CPAP in survival among severe OSA patients [12]. After 10 years of follow-up, severe OSA patients under CPAP treatment had an adjusted odds ratio for fatal cardiovascular mortality that did not differ significantly from non-OSA healthy individuals. The results suggest that treatment with CPAP for at least 4 hours per nights significantly reduces the raised cardiovascular risk reported in untreated severe OSA.

Summary

Many recent prospective, long-term, controlled studies suggest that in untreated patients with sleep apnea, the risk of death from all causes and particularly cardiovascular causes is increased. There is a relation between the severity of this disease and cardiovascular risk, but the effective treatment with nasal CPAP significantly reduces the mortality associated with this medical condition. Nevertheless, clinicians must go forward because of the research in the field. From a public health point this is a cost-effective investment, because CPAP treatment seems to decrease the excess health care costs for cardiovascular disease and car accidents incurred by OSA [49].

References

[1] Young T, Palta M, Dempsey J, et al. The occurrence of sleep-disordered breathing among middle-age adults. N Engl J Med 1993;328:1230–5.

[2] Duran J, Esnaola S, Rubio R, et al. Obstructive sleep apnoea-hypopnea and related clinical features in a population-based sample of subjects aged 30 to 70 yr. Am J Respir Crit Care Med 2001;163:685–9.

[3] Barbé F, Pericas J, Muñoz A, et al. Automobile accidents in patients with sleep apnea syndrome. Am J Respir Crit Care Med 1998;158:18–22.

[4] Teran-Santos J, Jimenez-Gomez A, Cordero-Guevara J. The association between sleep apnoea and the risk of traffic accidents. Cooperative Group Burgos-Santander. N Engl J Med 1999; 340:847–51.

[5] Stradling J. Con: sleep apnea does not cause cardiovascular disease. Am J Respir Crit Care Med 2004;169:148–9.

[6] Lavie P. Pro: sleep apnea causes cardiovascular disease. Am J Respir Crit Care Med 2004;169: 147–8.

[7] Sullivan CE, Issa F, Berthon-Jones M, et al. Reversal of obstructive sleep apnea by continuous positive airway pressure applied by the nares. Lancet 1981;1:862–5.

[8] Giles TL, Lasserson TJ, Smith BJ, et al. Continuous positive airways pressure for obstructive sleep apnoea in adults. Cochrane Database Syst Rev 2006;3:CD001106.

[9] Karlawish JHT, Pack AI. Addressing the ethical problems of randomized and placebo-controlled trials of CPAP. Am J Respir Crit Care Med 2001; 163:809–10.

[10] Cohn JN, Tognoni G. A randomized trial of the angiotensin receptor blocker valsartan in chronic heart failure. N Engl J Med 2001;345:1667–75.

[11] American Academy of Sleep Medicine. International classification of sleep disorders. Westchester (IL): AASM; 2005.

[12] Marin JM, Carrizo SJ, Vicente E, et al. Long-term cardiovascular outcomes in men with obstructive sleep apnoea-hypopnoea with or without treatment with continuous positive airway pressure: an observational study. Lancet 2005;365: 1046–53.

[13] Yaggi HK, Concato J, Kernan WN, et al. Obstructive sleep apnea as a risk factor for stroke and death. N Engl J Med 2005;353:2034–41.

[14] Arzt M, Young T, Finn L, et al. Association of sleep disordered breathing and the occurrence of stroke. Am J Respir Crit Care Med 2005;172: 1447–51.

[15] Concato J, Shah N, Horwitz RI. Randomized, controlled trials, observational studies, and the hierarchy of research designs. N Engl J Med 2000;342:1887–92.

[16] Benson K, Hartz AJ. A comparison of observational studies and randomized, controlled trials. N Engl J Med 2000;342:1878–86.

[17] Koenig S. Pulmonary complications of obesity. Am J Med Sci 2001;321:249–79.

[18] Ferretti A, Giampiccolo P, Cavalli A, et al. Expiratory flow limitation and orthopnea in massively obese subjects. Chest 2001;119:1401–8.

[19] Newman AB, Foster G, Givelber R, et al. Progression and regression of sleep-disordered breathing with changes in weight: the Sleep Heart Health Study. Arch Intern Med 2005;165: 2408–13.

[20] Yusuf S, Hawken S, Ounpuu S, et al. Obesity and the risk of myocardial infarction in 27,000 participants from 52 countries: a case-control study. Lancet 2005;366:1640–9.

[21] Vgontzas AN, Bixler EO, Chrousos GP. Sleep apnea is a manifestation of the metabolic syndrome. Sleep Med Rev 2005;9:211–24.

[22] Adams KF, Schazkin A, Harris T, et al. Overweight, obesity, and mortality in large prospective cohort of persons 50 to 71 years old. N Engl J Med 2006;355:763–78.

[23] Smith SC Jr, Blair SN, Bonow RO. AHA/ACC guidelines for preventing heart attack and death in patients with atherosclerotic cardiovascular disease: 2001 update—a statement for healthcare professionals from the American Heart Association and the American College of Cardiology. J Am Coll Cardiol 2001;38:1581–3.

[24] Romero-Corral A, Montori VM, Somers VK, et al. Association of bodyweight with total mortality and with cardiovascular events in coronary artery disease: a systematic review of cohort studies. Lancet 2006;368:666–78.

[25] Dyer AR, Stamler J, Garside DB, et al. Long-term consequences of body mass index for cardiovascular mortality: the Chicago Heart Association Detection Project in Industry study. Ann Epidemiol 2004;14:101–8.

[26] Pi-Sunyer FX. The obesity epidemic: pathophysiology and consequences of obesity. Obes Res 2002;10(Suppl 2):97–104.

[27] Krauss RM, Winston M, Fletcher BJ, et al. Obesity: impact on cardiovascular disease. Circulation 1998;98:1472–6.

[28] Shamsuzzaman AS, Gersh BJ, Somers VK. Obstructive sleep apnea: implications for cardiac and vascular disease. JAMA 2003;290:1906–14.

[29] Wright J, Johns R, Watt I, et al. Health effects of obstructive sleep apnoea and the effectiveness of continuous positive airways pressure: a systematic review of the research evidence. BMJ 1997; 314:851–60.

[30] He J, Kryger MH, Zorick FJ, et al. Mortality and apnea index in obstructive sleep apnea: experience in 385 male patients. Chest 1988;94:9–14.

[31] Gonzalez-Rothi RJ, Foresman GE, Block AJ. Do patient with sleep apnea die in their sleep? Chest 1988;94:531–8.

[32] Bliwise DL, Bliwise NG, Partinen M, et al. Sleep apnea and mortality in an aged cohort. Am J Public Health 1988;78:544–7.

[33] Ancoli-Israel S, Kripke DF, Klauber MR, et al. Morbidity, mortality and sleep-disordered breathing in community dwelling elderly. Sleep 1996;19:277–82.

[34] Mant A, King M, Saunders NA, et al. Four-year follow-up of mortality and sleep related respiratory disturbance in non-demented seniors. Sleep 1995;18:433–8.

[35] Lavie P, Hever P, Peled R, et al. Mortality in sleep apnea patients: a multivariate analysis of risk factors. Sleep 1995;18:149–57.

[36] Peker Y, Hedner J, Kraiczi H, et al. Respiratory disturbance index: an independent predictor of mortality in coronary artery disease. Am J Respir Crit Care Med 2000;162:81–6.

[37] Mooe T, Franklin KA, Holmström K, et al. Sleep-disordered breathing and coronary artery disease: long-term prognosis. Am J Respir Crit Care Med 2001;164:1910–3.

[38] Lavie P, Lavie L, Herer P. All-cause mortality in males with sleep apnoea syndrome: declining mortality rates with age. Eur Respir J 2005;25: 514–20.

[39] Hagenah GC, Gueven E, Andreas S. Influence of obstructive sleep apnoea in coronary artery disease: a 10-year follow-up. Respir Med 2006;100: 180–2.

[40] Marti S, Sampol G, Muñoz X, et al. Mortality in severe sleep apnea/hypopnea syndrome patients: impact of treatment. Eur Respir J 2002;20:1511–8.

[41] Marin JM, Gascon JM, Carrizo S, et al. Prevalence of sleep apnoea syndrome in the Spanish adult population. Int J Epidemiol 1997;26:381–6.

[42] The fifth report of the joint national committee on detection, evaluation, and treatment of high blood pressure. Arch Intern Med 1993;153: 154–83.

[43] Montserrat JM, Amilibia J, Barbe F, et al. Tratamiento del sindrome de las apneas-hipopneas durante el sueño. Arch Bronconeumol 1998;34: 204–6.

[44] Barbe F, Mayoralas LR, Duran J, et al. Treatment with continuous positive airway pressure is not effective in patients with sleep apnea but no daytime sleepiness: a randomized, controlled trial. Ann Intern Med 2001;134:1015–23.

[45] Krieger J, Meslier N, Lebrun T, et al. Accidents in obstructive sleep apnea patients treated with nasal continuous positive pressure: a prospective study. Chest 1997;112:1561–6.

[46] Keenan SP, Burt H, Ryan F, et al. Long-term survival of patients with obstructive sleep apnea treated by uvulopalatopharyngoplasty or nasal CPAP. Chest 1994;105:155–9.

[47] Campos-Rodriguez F, Peña-Griñan N, Reyes-Nuñez N, et al. Mortality in obstructive sleep apnea-hypopnea patients treated with positive airway pressure. Chest 2005;128:624–33.

[48] Doherty LS, Kiely JL, Swan V, et al. Long-term effects of nasal continuous positive airway pressure therapy on cardiovascular outcomes in sleep apnea syndrome. Chest 2005;127:2076–84.

[49] McNicholas WT, Bonsignore MR. Sleep apnoea as an independent risk factor for cardiovascular disease: current evidence, basic mechanism and research priorities. Eur Respir J 2007;29: 156–78.

SLEEP
MEDICINE
CLINICS

Sleep Med Clin 2 (2007) 603–613

ELSEVIER
SAUNDERS

Obstructive Sleep Apnea in Pregnancy

Fotis Kapsimalis, MD[a],*, Meir Kryger, MD, FRCCP[b]

The first report of sleep apnea in pregnancy, published in 1978 [1], raised concerns that snoring effects on alveolar ventilation and systemic arterial pressure could have adverse implications on maternal cardiorespiratory reserve and fetal heart rate and acid-base homeostasis. The concept that obstructive sleep apnea (OSA) in pregnancy can have negative health effects has been reinforced by the publication of several case reports of sleep-disordered breathing (SDB) during pregnancy [2].

The relationship between pregnancy and SDB is complex. Paradoxically, pregnancy leads to physical and biochemical changes that may both reduce and increase the risk for the development of sleep apnea [3,4]. The presence of OSA in pregnancy may have adverse effects on maternal and fetal outcomes [3–5].

This article reviews the alterations of sleep and pulmonary mechanics and patency of upper airways during pregnancy, the role of the female hormones, the risk factors and prevalence of SDB in pregnancy, the effects on maternal and fetal outcomes, and therapeutic and preventive strategies.

Alterations of sleep in normal pregnancy

Normal pregnancy is associated with changes in the sleep pattern and architecture starting in the first trimester. These changes are thought to be related to the increased levels of female reproductive hormones (estrogen and progesterone) that accompany pregnancy and to several physical phenomena that occur in pregnancy and may affect the normal

[a] Department of Thoracic Medicine, Sleep Laboratory, Henry Dunant Hospital, 107 Mesogeion Avenue, 115 26 Athens, Greece
[b] Gaylord Sleep Medicine, Gaylord Hospital, University of Connecticut, Gaylord Farm Road, Wallingford, CT 06942, USA
* Corresponding author.
E-mail address: fogeka@otenet.gr (F. Kapsimalis).

doi:10.1016/j.jsmc.2007.07.002

sleep-wakefulness cycle like nausea, vomiting, increased urinary frequency, heartburn, discomfort, bladder distention, and fetal movements [5,6]. Sleep alterations observed in normal pregnancy include the following:

> Subjective
> > Increased sleep duration
> > Increased awakenings
> > Insomnia
> > Sleep disturbance
> > Daytime sleepiness
> > Daily naps
> Objective
> > Increased total sleep time (first trimester)
> > Decreased sleep efficiency
> > Decreased stages 3 and 4 of non-REM sleep
> > Decreased REM sleep
> > Increased stage 1 of non-REM sleep
> > Increased wake time after sleep onset
> > Decreased total sleep time (third trimester)

During the first trimester, sleep duration, daytime sleepiness, and sleep disturbance caused by frequent awakenings and insomnia are increased [6,7]. Objective investigations with polysomnography (PSG) have shown an increase of total sleep time and a decrease of sleep efficiency and slow wave non–rapid eye movement (REM) sleep (stages 3 and 4) [8].

In the second trimester, the total nocturnal sleep time decreases to normal duration but sleep complaints increase resulting in nocturnal awakenings [6,7]. Slow wave sleep remains reduced, whereas REM sleep is slightly decreased [8,9].

During the third trimester, most women report sleep disturbances and nocturnal awakenings and daily naps [6,7,10]. The sleep architecture is altered with decreased total sleep time [8,9], increased wakening time after sleep onset [11,12], increased stage 1 of non-REM sleep [11], decreased stages 3 and 4 [8,10], and decreased REM sleep [8,9,11,12].

Respiration in pregnancy and risk of sleep-disordered breathing

The hormonal and anatomic changes of pregnancy affect respiratory function and gas exchange. Some of these changes could potentially induce the development of SDB, whereas other changes might be protective against SDB [3]. Physiologic changes related to sleep-disordered breathing during pregnancy include the following:

> Detrimental
> > Weight gain
> > Elevation of the diaphragm
> > Reduction of functional reserve capacity

> > Nasal congestion and rhinitis
> > Hyperventilation
> > Increased stage 1 of non-REM sleep
> > Sleep fragmentation
> Protective
> > Avoidance of supine position
> > Increased minute ventilation
> > Increased dilating actions of pharyngeal muscles
> > Reduction of REM sleep

Sleep-disordered breathing promoting mechanisms

Physical changes

Weight gain in pregnancy may predispose to SDB development as in the general population [13]. Although there are no prospective studies evaluating the effect of rate of the weight gain on breathing during sleep in pregnant women, most of the case reports of SDB in pregnancy involve obese women [1–3].

The elevation of the diaphragm from uterine enlargement during pregnancy results in a reduction in functional residual capacity, which is reduced during sleep because of postural effects on diaphragm mechanics [14]. Maternal oxygenation reserve is reduced in pregnancy because of increased alveolar-arterial oxygen gradient, decreased functional residual capacity, and increased airway closure above functional residual capacity during tidal ventilation resulting in ventilation-perfusion mismatch. These effects are more prominent in late pregnancy and in the supine position [14–17]. Mild supine hypoxemia has been observed during wakefulness and sleep in healthy pregnant women during the third trimester [17,18].

The increase of blood volume resulting in hyperemia and edema of the nasal mucosa can lead to nasal congestion in pregnancy. High estrogen levels may also cause vasomotor rhinitis, which is found in 20% of pregnancies in the third trimester [19]. It has been reported that 42% of women at 36 weeks gestation complain of nasal congestion and rhinitis [20]. Similar mechanisms may be responsible for the reduction of pharyngeal dimensions observed during pregnancy [21]. Reduced nasopharyngeal patency may promote the development of SDB in pregnancy [22].

Hormonal changes

The high circulating levels of progesterone and estrogen [23], required for pregnancy maintenance, influence ventilation in pregnant women. It is known that progesterone enhances respiratory drive resulting in hyperventilation, which leads to a reduction of arterial carbon dioxide pressure and respiratory alkalosis [24,25]. This may lead to instability of respiration and the development of central apneas during the transition from wakefulness to sleep in nonpregnant women, although this effect has not been investigated in pregnant women [26]. The increased stage 1 and sleep fragmentation from the frequent awakenings in the third trimester [11] may predispose pregnant women to an increased frequency of central apneas. The enhanced respiratory drive, however, may lead to more negative inspiratory pressures, increased suction pressure on upper airway structures, and a tendency for collapse of the upper airways during sleep [27].

Sleep-disordered breathing protective mechanisms

Physical changes

It is known that supine sleep posture may increase the frequency of OSA events compared with the lateral or prone positions [28]. Most pregnant women during late pregnancy prefer to sleep in lateral posture, which may prevent SDB. This posture also preserves cardiac output and oxygenation [29].

Obstructive events are more frequent during REM sleep when breathing is most unstable and women have more apneas and hypopneas during this stage of sleep [30]. The observed reduction of REM sleep during late pregnancy [11,12] may protect pregnant women from SDB.

Hormonal changes

The known increase of minute ventilation during pregnancy may serve as an adaptation to the increased oxygen consumption demands of pregnancy [25]. Progesterone stimulates respiratory drive directly or enhances the sensitivity of the respiratory center to CO_2, resulting in increased tidal volume and hyperventilation [24,31]. Although this action may potentially induce SDB in pregnancy, it could also be protective against SDB. The higher respiratory drive enhances responsiveness of upper airway dilator muscles to chemical stimuli during sleep and protects against upper airway occlusion [32]. It has been shown that progesterone increases the electromyographic activity of pharyngeal dilating muscles [33]. Although these studies have not been done in pregnant women, these actions of progesterone may potentially prevent SDB in pregnancy.

Obstructive sleep apnea and pregnancy

Hypoxia, sleep-disordered breathing, and normal pregnancy

Late pregnancy may be associated with decreased oxygenation in the supine position and there is concern that even mild respiratory disturbances during sleep may result in significant reduction of maternal and fetal oxygenation. Studies on maternal hypoxemia during sleep have conflicting results. Brownell and colleagues [34] in a study with PSG of six healthy pregnant women at 36 weeks gestation and postpartum found no nocturnal oxygen desaturation and a decreased index of apneas and hypopneas during pregnancy compared with the postpartum period. In contrast, Feinsilver and colleagues [35] studied 12 healthy pregnant women at late pregnancy and found lower basal oxygen saturation and higher frequency of desaturation episodes greater than 4% in comparison with 10 nonpregnant women. After delivery, nocturnal oxygenation returned to normal in seven women who were studied with sleep study. Only one pregnant woman had abnormal apnea-hypoxia index (AHI) of moderate severity. The authors suggested that the observed oxygen desaturation was not associated with SDB. Also, Hertz and colleagues [11] found a significant reduction of nocturnal oxygen saturation in 12 women in late pregnancy compared with postpartum nights. In a study of 13 nonpregnant women, 13 pregnant normotensive women, and 15 women with pregnancy-induced hypertension (PIH) at more than 35 weeks pregnancy, it was shown that mean arterial oxygen saturation (Sao_2) was lower in pregnant women compared with nonpregnant women. Three normotensive pregnant and four women with PIH spent more than 20% of total sleep time with Sao_2 less than 90% [18].

In a recent study of 21 women at 36 weeks of gestation the frequency of obstructive respiratory events was significantly lower during pregnancy than postpartum (5.81 ± 2.1 versus 12.1 ± 2.7 events per hour; $P < .001$) and level of oxygenation was lower in the supine position than in the sitting position [36]. It has also been reported that oxygen saturation during sleep was lower during pregnancy than postpartum but there was no correlation between levels of Sao_2 and apneas or hypopneas or the percentage of REM sleep [37].

Although during pregnancy in normal women oxygen desaturation is reduced in the supine position, there is not enough evidence to indicate that frequency of SDB is increased. Instead, there is evidence that healthy pregnant women are protected from the development of severe OSA. In a study of 10 women with multiple pregnancies in the third trimester it was found that arterial oxygen was well preserved and there were no obstructive events. Despite the alterations of the respiratory system by the large uterus there was no evidence of sleep apnea events [38].

Recent data suggest that normal pregnancy is not associated with precipitation of sleep apnea in nonobese women. Maasilta and colleagues [39] compared 11 obese pregnant women with 11 pregnant women of normal weight at early (12 weeks) and late pregnancy (30 weeks). In early pregnancy, AHI (1.7 versus 0.2 events per hour; $P < .05$) and oxygen desaturation more than 4% (5.3 versus 0.3 events per hour; $P < .005$) were higher in the obese group and increased slightly at late pregnancy. One obese mother with 6% of total sleep time spent with Sao_2 less than 90% had an infant with growth retardation. Although there was no development of clinically significant OSA, obese healthy women had marginal deterioration in their sleep respiration in comparison with women of normal weight. Obesity may predispose pregnant women to the development of SDB and be related to adverse pregnancy outcomes even without the presence of significant OSA.

Prevalence of obstructive sleep apnea in pregnancy

The prevalence of OSA during pregnancy is not known because there are no prospective large population-based epidemiologic studies addressing this issue. Over the last three decades, the association of OSA with pregnancy has been based on published case reports with only some of them having polysomnographic documentation of the sleep apnea syndrome [1,2,40–49].

The first report was published by Joel-Cohen and Schoenfeld [1] in 1978 and included three cases of pregnant women with clinically diagnosed OSA. They reported no maternal complication and intrauterine infant growth retardation in one case. The largest cohort was reported by Schoenfeld and colleagues [2] with eight cases of clinically diagnosed OSA, which all resulted in delivery of babies with low birth weight. PSG was not performed. All these women were obese with snoring and witnessed

apneas. Kowall and colleagues [40] reported a case of severe OSA (AHI of 78.6 events per hour) that was significantly improved at 12 weeks postpartum. In another report [41] an obese woman developed severe sleep apnea in the third trimester and her baby was born with growth retardation. At postpartum there was no improvement of sleep apnea.

Only eight cases [40,41,42,45–49] of documented OSA in pregnant women have been published in the literature. In the rest of the reports diagnosis of sleep apnea was made clinically. In five cases with documented OSA [40,42,45,46,49], the mother had PIH and one case reported severe pulmonary hypertension [44]. Intrauterine infant growth retardation was reported in three cases [41,46,49], whereas in two other cases infants had normal birth weight [42,45].

Edwards and colleagues [50] investigated 11 women who were referred for suspected SDB, at late pregnancy and 3 months following delivery, and found that AHI in non-REM and REM sleep (63 ± 15 versus 18 ± 4 events per hour; $P < .03$) and minimum nocturnal hemoglobin saturation ($86\% \pm 2\%$ versus $91\% \pm 1\%$; $P < .01$) were significantly improved after parturition. They also found that during pregnancy arterial blood pressure peaked at 180 mm in comparison with 140 mm Hg postnatally. This study indicates that late pregnancy may worsen the severity of SDB and lead to increased blood pressure.

These reports suggest that OSA may develop in women with risk factors for SDB or may worsen the severity of pre-existing OSA with several adverse outcomes, such as the development of maternal PIH or fetal intrauterine growth retardation. Table 1 presents published data on OSA during

Table 1: Published reports of OSA during pregnancy

Author	Number of cases	Method of diagnosis	Maternal complications	Fetal complications
Joel-Cohen and Schoenfeld [1]	3	Clinical	None	IUGR
Schoenfeld et al [2]	8	Clinical	None	IUGR
Conti et al [42]	1	PSG	PIH	None
Kowall et al [40]	1	PSG	PIH	NA
Hastie et al [43]	1	Clinical	DM	None
Charbonneau et al [41]	1	PSG	DM	IUGR
Sherer et al [45]	1	PSG	DM, PIH	None
Lefcourt and Rodis [46]	1	PSG	PIH	IUGR
Lewis et al [44]	1	Clinical	PH	None
Taibah et al [47]	1	PSG	Hypothyroidism	NA
Pieters et al [48]	1	PSG	None	None
Roush and Bell [49]	1	PSG	PIH	IUGR

Abbreviations: DM, diabetes mellitus; IUGR, intrauterine growth retardation; NA, not available; PIH, pregnancy-induced hypertension; PSG, polysomnography.

measurem
spite the r
tween SD]
causality [
changes ir
of preecla
ways in w
ratory flo
OSA is
has been
hypertens
has been
ing pregn
Moreover,
nocturnal
vous syst
[77], elev
stances [7
tive stress
vascular
supports
the devel
pregnant
duced an
oxidatior
mediates
eclampsia
ity of the
cardiovas
worsens
nal hypc
and vasc
emia and
may occ
SDB, hov
ment of
ever, wor
In a rec
women
with 10 [
tension
monitor
events v
The autl
damage
hemody
In a r
vestigate
dothelia
17 wom
nant co
by the r
lated th
pulse wa
Females
disturba
events p

pregnancy. Further studies with larger number of subjects and polysomnographic documented sleep apnea would better determine the true prevalence of OSA during pregnancy.

Risk factors for the development of obstructive sleep apnea during pregnancy

There is evidence that snoring is increased during pregnancy and is common in the third trimester. Snoring is not a specific symptom for the presence of OSA during pregnancy, although it has been shown that self-reported snoring correlates with objective findings of PSG [51].

Loube and colleagues [52], in an investigation of self-reported snoring during pregnancy, showed that 14% of 350 pregnant women at the second and third trimester reported habitual snoring in comparison with 4% of 110 nonpregnant controls. Shutte and colleagues [53] showed that 27% of normal women reported snoring at the last trimester of pregnancy.

A retrospective study with data obtained the day of delivery found that 23% of 502 pregnant women reported loud snoring in the last week of the third trimester, whereas only 4% reported loud snoring before pregnancy [54]. Snoring frequency was increased during the progression of pregnancy. Similarly, Hedman and colleagues [55] found an increase in the prevalence of habitual snoring from 5% before pregnancy to 10.4% during late pregnancy and a decrease of snoring to 4.4% at 3 months after delivery. In a recent retrospective study at postpartum, 45% of 438 women reported habitual snoring during pregnancy, whereas 85% of them were nonsnorers before pregnancy [56].

In a prospective study of 155 women investigating the presence and progression of SDB symptoms during pregnancy, Pien and colleagues [57] showed that not only snoring but also gasping, choking, and witnessed apneas were increased significantly during pregnancy suggesting that pregnant women are at high risk for the development of OSA syndrome. Although in most women the estimated probability of OSA syndrome remained low, it was speculated that 10% of subjects may develop significant sleep apnea during pregnancy. Although these symptoms are more specific for sleep apnea than snoring alone, the prediction of likelihood from the apnea symptom score has not been validated in pregnancy and the lack of polysomnographic evaluation cannot confirm this hypothesis.

The pathophysiologic mechanisms responsible for the increase in snoring during pregnancy remain unclear. Obesity is a major risk factor for sleep apnea in the general population and the increase of body weight is associated with the development of SDB symptoms [58]. During pregnancy,

increased initial body mass index and greater changes in neck circumference have been associated with higher prevalence of SDB symptoms [57]. In several studies women with habitual snoring during pregnancy were heavier at baseline than nonsnorers [39,54]. Franklin and colleagues [54] found that pregnant women who reported habitual snoring gained significantly more weight than nonsnorers suggesting that gestational weight gain may also be important to the development of snoring.

In the general population, it has been demonstrated that neck circumference is a predictor of the likelihood for sleep apnea, independent of weight [59]. Changes in neck circumference may reflect changes in upper airway anatomy during pregnancy. Recently, Izci and colleagues [60,61] demonstrated that upper airways are significantly narrower in pregnant women during late pregnancy in comparison with nonpregnant women or measurement in postpartum period. It has also been found that the upper airway of pregnant women was wider in the seated position in comparison with nonpregnant women in wakefulness but there was no difference in the supine position. This finding indicates a greater decrease in airway caliber on lying down in pregnant women [61]. The role of progesterone on increased pharyngeal dilator muscle activity in seated pregnant women may explain the wider airway caliber but there are no studies in pregnant women.

Mechanisms that explain narrowing of upper airways in pregnancy are not well elucidated. Several physiologic changes during pregnancy may predispose to upper airway increased resistance and reduced cross-sectional area. The weight gain in pregnancy [39,54], the abdominal mass loading, and elevation of the diaphragm result in reduced lung volumes and functional residual capacity and tracheal shortening leading to upper airway narrowing [14,16,61]. The pharyngeal edema of pregnancy and fat or soft tissue deposition [21,54,61] around upper airways can also lead to narrowing [57,62–64]. In a recent study, physical examination showed that snoring pregnant women had abnormal oropharyngeal anatomy and nasal mucosa engorgement [64]. Sleep deprivation and fragmentation in pregnancy [11,12] may also lead to loss of dilating muscle activity [65], and increased upper airway collapsibility [66] results in this further upper airway narrowing, although there are no similar studies during pregnancy.

Obesity and narrowing of the upper airway in the supine position could explain the increased prevalence of snoring in pregnant women. Bradley and colleagues [67] have reported that snorers have narrower upper airways than nonsnorers of 325 pregnant women did not find a relationship between snoring and infant birth weight. The lack of PSG documentation of sleep apnea and methodologic limitations of these studies offer only preliminary evidence of the possible relationship between OSA and fetal adverse outcomes. It has been reported that nonapneic snorers may not have nocturnal hypoxemia [86]. Adequate oxygen delivery and protection against transient nocturnal desaturation during pregnancy may be enhanced, however, by the high oxygen carrying capacity of the fetal hemoglobin and the high uptake and delivery of the fetal circulation [17]. The potential link between SDB, oxidative stress, endothelial dysfunction, and the development of PIH may affect placental and fetal development, however, with possible fetal complications.

Treatment and prevention strategies

Treatment of sleep-disordered breathing during pregnancy

Efforts to treat SDB are of paramount importance during pregnancy because of the possible adverse effects on pregnancy outcome and fetal health. In documented OSA syndrome, treatment is especially indicated in the presence of maternal nocturnal hypoxemia [5]. Treatment includes conservative measures (see next) and the application of CPAP by nasal mask [87]. Oral appliances have not been investigated in pregnancy-related SDB and they are not suggested because they could be impractical [3,46]. Surgical therapies like uvulopalatopharyngoplasty are not recommended during pregnancy because they are less effective and they have increased risk for complications during pregnancy [3,87]. Similarly, tracheostomy has been reported in one case but it is rarely necessary [43].

Conservative measures include control of body weight gain, avoidance of sleep time spent in the supine position, elevation of the head during sleep, and restriction of alcohol and sedatives consumption [87]. These general measures are useful even in non-OSA syndrome pregnant women who report increases of simple snoring or daytime sleepiness without the documentation of sleep apneas [5].

In the presence of significant OSA syndrome or significant SDB-related nocturnal hypoxemia, nasal CPAP is the therapy of choice [3–5]. It has been suggested that CPAP may lower cardiac output [88], but this reduction is not clinically significant in subjects with normal cardiac function or in pregnancy-induced physiologic hypervolemia [3,5]. The use of CPAP during pregnancy has been shown to be safe, effective, and well tolerated [40,42,44,49,64,73,89]. In a study on preeclampsia [73], CPAP has been reported to abolish inspiratory flow limitation and lower the mean nocturnal blood pressure. Given the lack of enough evidence, CPAP therapy is not recommended in preeclampsia without objective documentation of sleep apnea [3].

Although supplemental oxygen therapy has been suggested in therapy of OSA syndrome during pregnancy [5], it may prolong apnea duration and lead to hypercapnia and its effectiveness remain unclear [90]. It should be considered only in pregnant women who are unable to tolerate CPAP [3].

Prevention of sleep-disordered breathing during pregnancy

Because of the possible adverse outcomes associated with SDB during pregnancy, efforts should be made for recognition of pregnant women at risk for the development of SDB. Every pregnant woman should be questioned about the symptoms suggesting OSA (snoring, observed apnea, daytime sleepiness) and if apnea is likely should be evaluated with full overnight PSG. Although there are no guidelines or consensus regarding the management of pregnancy-induced SDB, indications for PSG could be expanded according to the current evidence of the relationship between SDB and pregnancy [5]. The authors suggest that pregnant women who develop PIH or preeclampsia (particularly if they are obese) should be candidates for comprehensive PSG [3,5]. In addition, those with a history of previous babies with intrauterine growth retardation or persistent sleep-related symptoms associated with snoring or obesity should be further evaluated [5]. Finally, after delivery, women with proved SDB developed during pregnancy with persistent symptoms and weight retention should be further evaluated for the presence of remaining SDB. Subjects with known OSA should be reevaluated after weight loss to titrate maintenance therapy. Women with sleep apnea during pregnancy should be closely monitored for recurrence in subsequent pregnancies [3].

Summary

During pregnancy several physical and hormonal alterations may affect normal sleep and the respiratory system and predispose pregnant women to the development of SDB or worsen pre-existing OSA syndrome. Current data suggest that the incidence of snoring is increased during pregnancy, but the exact incidence and prevalence of OSA syndrome in pregnancy remains uncertain and needs to be investigated in epidemiologic studies. SDB has been associated with several complications of pregnancy affecting maternal and fetal health. Clinicians should evaluate more closely obese pregnant women and those who develop hypertension. Early recognition and treatment of SDB may improve the outcome of pregnancy but the indications for treatment of OSA syndrome need to be investigated [91]. The diagnosis of OSA syndrome in pregnancy requires a high index of suspicion and prevention of suspected SDB should be incorporated in the management of pregnancy.

References

[1] Joel-Cohen SJ, Schoenfeld A. Fetal response to periodic sleep apnea: a new syndrome in obstetrics. Eur J Obstet Gynecol Reprod Biol 1978;8(2):77–81.

[2] Schoenfeld A, Ovadia Y, Neri A, et al. Obstructive sleep apnea (OSA)-implications in maternal-fetal medicine: a hypothesis. Med Hypotheses 1989;30(1):51–4.

[3] Pien GW, Schwab RJ. Sleep disorders in pregnancy. Sleep 2004;27(7):1405–17.

[4] Edwards N, Middleton PG, Blyton DM, et al. Sleep disordered breathing and pregnancy. Thorax 2002;57:555–8.

[5] Santiago JR, Nolledo MS, Kinzler W, et al. Sleep and sleep disorders in pregnancy. Ann Intern Med 2001;134:396–408.

[6] Schweiger MS. Sleep disturbance in pregnancy: a subjective survey. Am J Obstet Gynecol 1972;114:879–82.

[7] Suzuki S, Dennerstein L, Greenwood KM, et al. Sleeping patterns during pregnancy in Japanese women. J Psychosom Obstet Gynaecol 1994;15:19–26.

[8] Lee KA, Zafke ME, McEnany G. Parity and sleep patterns during and after pregnancy. Obstet Gynecol 2000;95:14–8.

[9] Driver HS, Shapiro CM. A longitudinal study of sleep stages in young women during pregnancy and postpartum. Sleep 1992;15:449–53.

[10] Karakan I, Wayne H, Harman AW, et al. Characteristics of sleep patterns during late pregnancy and the postpartum periods. Am J Obstet Gynecol 1968;101:579–86.

[11] Hertz G, Fast A, Feinsilver S, et al. Sleep in normal late pregnancy. Sleep 1992;115:929–35.

[12] Bruner DP, Munch M, Biedermann K, et al. Changes in sleep and sleep electroencephalogram during pregnancy. Sleep 1994;17:576–82.

[13] Peppard PE, Young T, Palta M, et al. Longitudinal study of moderate weight change and sleep disordered breathing. JAMA 2000;284:3015–21.

[14] Weinberger SE, Weiss ST, Cohen WR, et al. State of the art: pregnancy and the lung. Am Rev Respir Dis 1980;121:559–81.

[15] Knuttgen HG, Emerson K. Physiological response to pregnancy at rest and during exercise. Aust N Z J Obstet Gynaecol 1974;3:365–7.

[16] Craig DB, Toole MA. Airway closure in pregnancy. Can Anaesth Soc J 1975;22:665–72.

[17] Awe RJ, Nicorta MB, Newsom TD, et al. Arterial oxygen and alveolar-arterial gradients in term pregnancy. Obstet Gynecol 1979;53:182–6.

[18] Bourne T, Ogilvy AJ, Vickers R, et al. Nocturnal hypoxemia in late pregnancy. Br J Anaesth 1995;75:678–82.

[19] Mabry RL. Rhinitis in pregnancy. South Med J 1986;79:965–71.

[20] Bende M, Gredmark T. Nasal stuffiness during pregnancy. Laryngoscope 1999;109:1108–10.

[21] Pilkington S, Carli F, Dakin MJ, et al. Increase in Mallampati score during pregnancy. Br J Anaesth 1995;74:638–42.

[22] Haponik EF, Smith PL, Bohlman ME, et al. Computerized tomography in obstructive sleep apnea: correlation of airway size with physiology during sleep. Am Rev Respir Dis 1983;127:221–6.

[23] Liou JH, Redar RW. Endocrinology in pregnancy. In: Creasy PK, Resnik R, editors. Maternal-fetal medicine. 4th edition. Philadelphia: Saunders; 1999. p. 379–91.

[24] White DP, Douglas NJ, Pickett CK, et al. Sexual influence in the control of breathing. J Appl Physiol 1983;54:874–9.

[25] Contreras G, Gutierrez M, Beroiza T, et al. Ventilatory drive and respiratory muscle function in pregnancy. Am Rev Respir Dis 1991;144:837–41.

[26] Skatrud JB, Dempsey JA. Interaction of sleep state and chemical stimuli in sustaining rhythmic ventilation. J Appl Physiol 1983;55:813–22.

[27] Remmers JE, deGroot WJ, Sauerland EK, et al. Pathogenesis of upper airway occlusion during sleep. J Appl Physiol 1978;44:931–8.

[28] Itasaka Y, Miyazaki S, Ishikawa K, et al. The influence of sleep position and obesity on sleep apnea. Psychiatry Clin Neurosci 2000;54:340–1.

[29] Mills GH, Chaffe AG. Sleeping positions adopted by pregnant women of more than 30 weeks gestation. Anaesthesia 1994;49:249–50.

[30] O'Connor C, Thornley KS, Hanly PJ. Gender differences in the polysomnographic features in obstructive sleep apnea. Am J Respir Crit Care Med 2000;161:1465–72.

[31] Prowse CM, Gaensler EA. Respiratory and acid-base changes during pregnancy. Anesthesiology 1965;26:381–92.

[32] Wheatley JR, White DP. The influence of sleep on pharyngeal reflexes. Sleep 1993;16:587–9.

[33] Popovic RM, White DP. Upper airway muscle activity in normal women: influence of hormonal status. J Appl Physiol 1998;84:1055–62.

[34] Brownell LG, West P, Kryger MH. Breathing during sleep in normal pregnant women. Am Rev Respir Dis 1986;133:38–41.

[35] Feinsilver SH, Hertz G, Albertario C, et al. Oxygen desaturation and sleep disordered breathing in normal pregnancy. Sleep Research 1991;20:378.

[36] Prodromakis E, Trakada G, Tsapanos V, et al. Arterial oxygen tension during sleep in the third trimester of pregnancy. Acta Obstet Gynecol Scand 2004;83(2):159–64.

[37] Trakada G, Tsapanos V, Spiropoulos K. Normal pregnancy and oxygenation during sleep. Eur J Obstet Gynecol Reprod Biol 2003;109(2): 128–32.

[38] Nikkola E, Ekblad U, Ekholm E, et al. Sleep in multiple pregnancy: breathing patterns, oxygenation, and periodic leg movements. Am J Obstet Gynecol 1996;174:1622–5.

[39] Maasilta P, Bachour A, Teramo K, et al. Sleep-related disordered breathing during pregnancy in obese women. Chest 2001;120:1448–54.

[40] Kowall J, Clark G, Nino Murcia G, et al. Precipitation of obstructive sleep apnea during pregnancy. Obstet Gynecol 1989;74:453–5.

[41] Charbonneau M, Falcone T, Cosio MG, et al. Obstructive sleep apnea in pregnancy: therapy and implications for fetal health. Am Rev Respir Dis 1991;144:461–3.

[42] Conti M, Izzo V, Muggiasca ML, et al. Sleep apnea syndrome in pregnancy: a case report. Eur J Anaesthesiol 1988;5(2):151–4.

[43] Hastie SJ, Prowse K, Peks WH, et al. Obstructive sleep apnoea during pregnancy requiring tracheostomy. Aust N Z J Obstet Gynaecol 1989;29: 365–7.

[44] Lewis DF, Chesson LF, Edwards MS, et al. Obstructive sleep apnea during pregnancy resulting in pulmonary hypertension. South Med J 1988; 91(8):761–2.

[45] Sherer DM, Caverly CB, Abramowicz JS. Severe obstructive sleep apnea and associated snoring documented during external topography. Am J Obstet Gynecol 1991;165:1300–1.

[46] Lefcourt LA, Rodis JF. Obstructive sleep apnea in pregnancy. Obstet Gynecol Surv 1996;51(8): 503–6.

[47] Taibah K, Ahmed M, Baessa E, et al. An unusual cause of obstructive sleep apnea presenting during pregnancy. J Laryngol Otol 1998;112: 1189–91.

[48] Pieters T, Amy JJ, Burrini D, et al. Normal pregnancy in primary alveolar hypoventilation treated with nocturnal nasal intermittent positive pressure ventilation. Eur Respir J 1995;8: 1424–7.

[49] Roush SF, Bell L. Obstructive sleep apnea in pregnancy. J Am Board Fam Pract 2004;17(4):292–4.

[50] Edwards N, Blyton DM, Hennesy A, et al. Severity of sleep disordered breathing improves following parturition. Sleep 2005;28(6):737–41.

[51] Bliwise DL, Nekich JC, Dement WC. Relative validity of self-reported snoring as symptoms of sleep apnea on a sleep clinic population. Chest 1991;99:600–8.

[52] Loube DI, Poceta JS, Morales MC, et al. Self-reported snoring in pregnancy: association with fetal outcome. Chest 1996;109:885–9.

[53] Schutte S, Del Conte A, Gross A, et al. Self-reported snoring and sleep in high risk pregnancies. Sleep Research 1995;24:342.

[54] Franklin KA, Holmgren PA, Jonsson F, et al. Snoring, pregnancy-induced hypertension and growth retardation of the fetus. Chest 2000; 117:137–41.

[55] Hedman C, Pohjasvaara T, Tolonen U, et al. Effects of pregnancy on mothers' sleep. Sleep Med 2002;3:37–42.

[56] Calaora-Tournadre D, Ragot S, Meurice JC, et al. [Obstructive sleep apnea syndrome during pregnancy: prevalence of main symptoms and relationship with pregnancy-induced hypertension and intra-uterine growth retardation]. Rev Med Interne 2006;27:291–5 [in French].

[57] Pien GW, Fife D, Pack AI, et al. Changes in symptoms of sleep disordered breathing during pregnancy. Sleep 2005;28(10):1299–305.

[58] Young T, Peppard PE, Gotlieb DJ. Epidemiology of obstructive sleep apnea: a population health perspective. Am J Respir Crit Care Med 2002; 165:1217–39.

[59] Davies RJ, Ali NJ, Stradling JR. Neck circumference and other clinical features in the diagnosis of the obstructive sleep apnea syndrome. Thorax 1992;47:101–5.

[60] Izci B, Vennelle M, Liston WA, et al. Sleep disordered breathing and upper airway size in pregnancy and postpartum. Eur Respir J 2006;27: 321–7.

[61] Izci B, Riha R, Martin SE, et al. The upper airway in pregnancy and pre-eclampsia. Am J Respir Crit Care Med 2003;167:137–40.

[62] Mohsenin V. Gender differences in the expression of sleep disordered breathing: the role of upper airway dimensions. Chest 2001;120: 1442–7.

[63] Schwab RJ, Gefter WB, Pack AI, et al. Dynamic imaging of the upper airways during respiration in normal subjects. J Appl Physiol 1993;74: 1504–14.

[64] Guilleminault C, Kreutzer M, Chang JL. Pregnancy, sleep disordered breathing and treatment with nasal continuous positive airway pressure. Sleep Med 2004;5:43–51.

[65] Leiter JC, Knuth SL, Bartlett D Jr. The effect of sleep deprivation on activity of the genioglossus muscle. Am Rev Respir Dis 1985;132:1242–5.

[66] Series F, Roy N, Marc I. Effects of sleep deprivation and sleep fragmentation on upper airway collapsibility in normal subjects. Am J Respir Crit Care Med 1994;150:481–5.

[67] Bradley TD, Brown IG, Grossman RF, et al. Pharyngeal size in snorers, nonsnorers, and patients with obstructive sleep apnea. N Engl J Med 1986; 315:1327–31.

[68] Zhang J, Zeisler J, Hatch MC, et al. Epidemiology of pregnancy induced hypertension. Epidemiol Rev 1997;19:218–32.

[69] Dekker GA, Sibai BM. Etiology and pathogenesis of preeclampsia: current concepts. Am J Obstet Gynecol 1998;179:1359–75.

[70] Redman CW, Berlin LJ, Bonnar J. Reversed diurnal blood pressure rhythm in hypertensive pregnancies. Clin Sci Mol Med Suppl 1976;3: 687s–9s.

[71] Guilleminault C, Querra-Salva M, Chowdhuri S, et al. Normal pregnancy, daytime sleepiness, snoring and blood pressure. Sleep Med 2000;1: 289–97.

[72] Wilcox I, Grunstein RR, Colins FL, et al. Circadian rhythm of blood pressure in patients with obstructive sleep apnea. Blood Press 1992;1:219–22.

[73] Edwards N, Blyton DM, Kirjavainen T, et al. Nasal pressure positive airway pressure reduces sleep-induced blood pressure increments in preeclampsia. Am J Respir Crit Care Med 2000;162:252–7.

[74] Connolly G, Razak ARA, Hayanga A, et al. Inspiratory flow limitation during sleep in preeclampsia: comparison with normal pregnant and nonpregnant women. Eur Respir J 2001;18:672–6.

[75] Peppard PE, Young T, Palta M, et al. Prospective study of the association between sleep-disordered breathing and hypertension. N Engl J Med 2000;342:1378–84.

[76] Fletcher EC. Invited review. Physiological consequences of intermittent hypoxia: systemic blood pressure. J Appl Physiol 2001;90:1600–5.

[77] Carlson JT, Rangemark C, Hedner JA. Attenuated endothelium-dependent vascular relaxation in patients with sleep apnea. J Hypertens 1996;14: 577–84.

[78] Phillips BG, Narkiewicz K, Pesek CA, et al. Effects of obstructive sleep apnea on endothelin-1 and blood pressure. J Hypertens 1999;17:61–6.

[79] Schulz R, Mahmoudi S, Hattar K, et al. Enhanced release of superoxide from polymorphonuclear neutrophils in obstructive sleep apnea: impact of continuous positive airway pressure therapy. Am J Respir Crit Care Med 2000;162:566–70.

[80] Walsh SW. Maternal-placental interactions of oxidative stress and antioxidants in preeclampsia. Semin Reprod Endocrinol 1998;16:93–104.

[81] Rodie VA, Freeman DJ, Sattar N, et al. Preeclampsia and cardiovascular disease: metabolic syndrome of pregnancy? Atherosclerosis 2004;175: 189–202.

[82] Edwards N, Blyton DM, Kirjavainen TT, et al. Hemodynamic responses to obstructive respiratory events during sleep are augmented in women with preeclampsia. Am J Hypertens 2001;14: 1090–5.

[83] Yinon D, Lowenstein L, Suraya S, et al. Preeclampsia is associated with sleep-disordered breathing and endothelial dysfunction. Eur Respir J 2006;27:328–33.

[84] Ritchie K. The fetal response to changes in the composition of maternal inspired air in human pregnancy. Semin Perinatol 1980;4:295–9.

[85] Gozal D, Reeves SR, Row BW, et al. Respiratory effects of gestational intermittent hypoxia in the developing rat. Am J Respir Crit Care Med 2003;167:1540–7.

[86] Hoffstein V. Snoring and nocturnal oxygenation. is there a relationship? Chest 1995;108:370–4.

[87] Feinsilver S, Hertz G. Respiration during pregnancy. Clin Chest Med 1992;13:637–44.

[88] Leech JA, Ascah KJ. Hemodynamic effects of nasal CPAP examined by Doppler echocardiography. Chest 1991;99:323–6.

[89] Polo O, Ekholm E. Nocturnal hypoventilation in pregnancy: reversal with nasal continuous positive airway pressure. Am J Obstet Gynecol 1995;173:238–9.

[90] Fletcher EC, Munafo DA. Role of nocturnal oxygen therapy in obstructive sleep apnea. When should it be used? Chest 1990;98:1497–504.

[91] Sahota PK, Jain SS, Dhand R. Sleep disorders in pregnancy. Curr Opin Pulm Med 2003;9(6): 477–83.

ELSEVIER
SAUNDERS

SLEEP
MEDICINE
CLINICS

Sleep Med Clin 2 (2007) 615–621

Prevalence and Impact of Central Sleep Apnea in Heart Failure

Patrick Lévy, MD, PhD[a,b],*, Jean-Louis Pépin, MD, PhD[a,b],
Renaud Tamisier, MD, PhD[a,b], Yannick Neuder, MD[c],
Jean-Philippe Baguet, MD, PhD[c], Shahrokh Javaheri, MD[d]

- Pathophysiologic consequences of sleep apnea and hypopnea
- Impact of CSA on mortality
- Summary
- References

Considering its medical, social, and economic consequences, congestive heart failure (CHF) is a growing major health issue [1,2]. Nearly 5 million Americans today have CHF, with a prevalence approaching 10 per 1,000 among people older than 65 years. In Europe, several studies in people over 45 years have shown that the prevalence of CHF varies from 0.5% in younger people to 16% in people over 75 years [3,4]. Medications, mainly β-blockers and biventricular pacing, coronary bypass surgery, and the use of multidisciplinary teams to treat heart failure have been shown to reduce the rate of hospitalizations, improve functional status, and reduce mortality [5–8]. However, heart failure continues to confer a worse prognosis than most cancers, with 1-year mortality of about 15% to 40% [5,6,8–10], depending on severity. Thus, factors that can contribute to the progression of heart failure and impair its prognosis are actively being researched.

Sleep breathing disorders are common in CHF, and the pathophysiology of the two conditions is closely linked. The need to identify and treat specifically such disorders for improving CHF is being actively sought. Periodic breathing with central sleep apnea (Hunter-Cheyne–Stokes or HCSB-CSA) occurs in 30% to 80% of patients with advanced CHF [11–14]. This breathing pattern is characterized by the presence of central apneas, with crescendo–decrescendo changes in tidal volume. HCSB has been associated with elevations of sympathetic nervous activity, which is an important predictor of CHF progression, arrhythmias, and mortality. Indeed, a few studies, but not all, have shown that CSA is a predictor of mortality of heart failure patients [15–19]. The objective of this article is to provide an overview of the prevalence and consequences of central sleep apnea in the context of CHF.

Prevalence of sleep apnea in heart failure patients varies greatly (Table 1). The variability depends on

a Inserm ERI 17, Hypoxia Pathophysiology (HP2) Laboratory, Joseph Fourier University, Grenoble, France
b Sleep Laboratory, EFCR, Pôle Rééducation et Physiologie, Centre Hospitalier Universitaire de Grenoble, Grenoble, France
c Cardiology and Hypertension Clinics, Centre Hospitalier Universitaire de Grenoble, Grenoble, France
d Sleepcare Diagnostics, 4780 Socialville-Fosters Road, Mason, OH 45040, USA
* Corresponding author: Pôle Rééducation et Physiologie, Centre Hospitalier Universitaire de Grenoble, Grenoble, France.
E-mail address: plevy@chu-grenoble.fr (P. Lévy).

1556-407X/07/$ – see front matter © 2007 Elsevier Inc. All rights reserved.
sleep.theclinics.com
doi:10.1016/j.jsmc.2007.08.001

Table 1:   Prevalence of sleep apnea in recent (2006–2007) prospective studies of systolic heart failure

Country (y) (Ref)	N	% AHI ≥ 10/hr	% AHI ≥ 15/hr	% CSA	% OSA	% β blockers
United States (06) [22]	100		49	37	12	10
New Zealand (05) [24]	56	68		15	53	30
China (07) [28]	126	71		46	25	80
UK (07) [27]	55		53	38	15	78
Germany (07) [26]	700		52	33	19	85
Germany (07) [25]	203	71		28	43	90

Abbreviations: AHI, apnea-hypopnea index; N, number; OSA, obstructive sleep apnea.

multiple factors, including whether the study is retrospective (referral bias), the threshold of apnea-hypopnea index (AHI) used to define the presence of clinically significant sleep disorder (disorder is threshold dependent), use of EEG to accurately define AHI per hour of sleep (in contrast to defining AHI per hour of recording time in the absence of EEG), and definition of hypopnea (use of 2%, 3%, or 4%, and arousals if EEG is available to define hypopnea). Similarly, the prevalence of CSA versus obstructive sleep apnea (OSA) also varies, depending on presence of obesity and snoring in the enrolled patients. Another important confounding issue is differentiation of obstructive and central hypopnea from each other, and this very much depends on the scorer. In spite of these issues, the prevalence of sleep apnea is alarmingly high in systolic heart failure.

Javaheri and colleagues [20], in a prospective longitudinal study, reported a prevalence (AHI equal to or greater than 15 per hour) of about 50% in stable subjects with systolic heart failure (mean left ventricular failure ejection fraction or LVEF) of 25%. Forty percent were reported to have CSA. A small study by Lanfranchi and colleagues [21] also demonstrated a high prevalence of HCSB (55%) in 47 subjects with LVEF less than 40%. A large retrospective study included 450 subjects with CHF, and reported a prevalence (AHI equal to or greater than 15 per hour) of 61%, and a 32% and 29% prevalence of OSA and CSA, respectively [13]. The high prevalence of OSA in the latter study [13] may be explained by the retrospective nature (the selection of the subjects), the size of the sample, and the criteria used to score hypopnea.

More recently, Javaheri [22] updated his results of 100 of 114 consecutive eligible patients with heart failure and LVEF less than 45% (see Table 1). Forty-nine percent of patients had at least moderate degree of sleep apnea (AHI greater than or equal to 15 per hour) with an average index of 49 per hour. Thirty-seven percent of patients had CSA and 12% had OSA. When comparing patients with CSA to those without sleep apnea, the markers associated with CSA were poorer functional classification, atrial fibrillation, $PaCO_2$ less than 36 mm Hg, LVEF less than 20%, and nocturnal ventricular arrhythmias, including more than 30 PVCs, more than one couplet, and more than one episode of ventricular tachycardia per hour. In contrast, when comparing heart failure patients with CSA to OSA, OSA patients were significantly more obese (mean body weight 109 kg plus or minus 27 kg versus 78 kg plus or minus 18 kg) and had habitual snoring (83% versus 38%). Javaheri thus concluded that hallmarks of CSA are Class III New York Heart Association (NYHA), atrial fibrillation, frequent nocturnal ventricular arrhythmias, low arterial PCO_2, and LVEF less than 20%.

In Javaheri's study, 10% of the patients were on β-blockers. One critical and highly discussed question is whether prevalence of CSA remains high in the face of newest treatments of heart failure. The possibility exists that use of β-blockers has reduced the prevalence of CSA. In this regard, the Canadian continuous positive airway pressure (CPAP) trial to treat patients with CSA and heart failure was stopped partly owing to the reduced rate of inclusion, compared with what was expected. Among the possible explanations, between 1998 when starting the study and 2004 when it was stopped, was the rate of use of both β-blockers and spironolactone, which was higher (86% versus 58%, respectively) [23]. The subjects were therefore being recruited as modern therapy of heart failure was evolving, during transition of improving cardiac function, which is known to improve CSA. The observation (falling prevalence of CSA) was therefore not surprising. In a study of a small number of stable CHF subjects [24], 53 of 87 eligible outpatients, predominantly male (77%) with mean LVEF of 34 plus or minus 9%, sleep disordered breathing (SDB) was demonstrated in 36 subjects (68%), including two subgroups: OSA (n = 28, 53%) and CSA (n = 8, 15%). The high prevalence of OSA and low prevalence of CSA in this study [24] was at least in part because of recruitment of subjects with higher LVEF than other studies. As noted elsewhere [13,22], CSA is more prevalent in individuals with low ejection fraction than individuals with OSA. As noted, in this study [24], the main LVEF was 34%.

Meanwhile, more recent studies of a large number of patients with systolic heart failure on contemporary therapy for heart failure show a high prevalence of CSA (see Table 1). A multicenter study from Germany [25] involved 203 CHF subjects who were stable in NYHA classes II and III and had a LVEF less than 40%. Polygraphy (without EEG) was used to record sleep studies. Data were centrally analyzed. Subject enrollment was irrespective of sleep-related symptoms. The majority of subjects were hospitalized and of male gender, mean age was 65 years. Seventy-one percent had an AHI of more than 10 per hour (n = 145), OSA occurred in 43% (n = 88), and Cheyne-Stokes respiration in 28% (n = 57) [25]. Another German study [26] involved 700 subjects with CHF (NYHA class greater than or equal to II, LVEF less than or equal to 40%). Treatment included angiotensin-converting enzyme-inhibitors or AT1-receptor blockers in 94%, diuretics in 87%, β-blockers in 85%, digitalis in 61%, and spironolactone in 62% of the subjects. Polygraphy (without EEG) SDB was used for diagnosis. Sleep apnea was present in 76% of the subjects (40% CSA and 36% OSA). CSA subjects were more symptomatic (NYHA class 2.9 plus or minus 0.5 versus no SDB 2.57 plus or minus 0.5, or OSA 2.57 plus or minus 0.5; $P<.05$) and had a lower LVEF (27 plus or minus 7% versus 29 plus or minus 3%; $P<.05$) than OSA subjects, confirming the result of previous studies [11,22].

Two other studies, one from United Kingdom, by Vazir and colleagues [27], and the other from China, by Zhao and colleagues [28], show high prevalence of central sleep apnea in spite of judicious use of β-blockers (see Table 1).

In summary, therefore, many studies show a high prevalence of sleep apnea in patients with systolic heart failure, making it the most common risk factor for sleep apnea. Furthermore, in spite of use β-blockers, prevalence of CSA remains quite high in this population.

Prevalence of sleep apnea in patients with a pace maker has been investigated in a multicenter study in eleven centers in Europe [30]. There were three different conditions leading to pace maker implantation: sinus node dysfunction, atrio-ventricular block, and heart failure. The prevalence of sleep-disordered breathing was very high, over 50% in all three groups. There was no correlation with age, body mass index, or symptoms such as excessive daytime sleepiness. Moreover, SDB were nearly exclusively obstructive in nature, even in the CHF group. Lastly, the prevalence was lower in this specific subgroup when compared with the two others: that is, sinus node dysfunction and atrio-ventricular block.

Although cardiac resynchronization therapy (CRT) may improve CSA, residual periodic breathing persists. CRT is usually indicated for heart failure patients with ventricular conduction delay, QRS greater than or equal to 130 ms, moderate to severe heart failure (NYHA class III or IV), LVEF less than or equal to 35%, and still symptomatic despite optimal medical treatment [31,32]. An early report of a few patients suggested that CRT was effective in suppressing CSA [33]. However, this has not been the case in the experience of the authors, and in a recent study [34] in which 77 heart failure subjects eligible for CRT were screened for the presence of SDB before and after CRT initiation (5.3 plus or minus 3 months), CSA was present in 36 (47%) and OSA in 26 (34%) of the subjects. CRT improved clinical and hemodynamic parameters. SDB parameters improved in CSA subjects only (AHI 31 plus or minus 16 per hour to 17 plus or minus 14 per hour; $P<.001$). After classifying short term clinical and hemodynamic CRT effects, improved SDB parameters in CSA occurred in responders only [34]. Residual central events after CRT are thus not rare and this is currently being studied in a large multicenter study conducted in Europe.

Pathophysiologic consequences of sleep apnea and hypopnea

There are a number of immediate and long-term pathophysiologic consequences of sleep apnea and hypopnea (Fig. 1). Immediate consequences of periodic breathing include hypoxemia and reoxygenation, hypercapnia and hypocapnia, and negative swings of intrathoracic pressure. These changes result in neurohormonal activation, release of inflammatory mediators, increases in transmural cardiac chambers, diminished oxygen delivery, and a host of other adverse effects reviewed elsewhere [35–39]. Regarding sympathetic activity, CSA has been shown to be associated with increased plasma and urinary excretion of norepinephrine, and also increased sympathetic activity of the vascular bed. This increase in muscle sympathetic nerve activity (MSNA) has been shown in nine patients with CHF [40]. HCSB increased MSNA burst frequency (from 45 plus or minus 5 bursts per minute during normal breathing to 50 plus or minus 5 bursts per minute during HCSB; $P<.05$) and total integrated nerve activity (to 117 plus or minus 7%; $P<.05$) [40]. The increase in MSNA was also proportional to the duration of HCSB, with higher values when HCSB was persistent versus intermittent. In addition, MSNA was higher during the second half of each apnea (increasing to 152 plus or minus 14%; $P<.01$) and

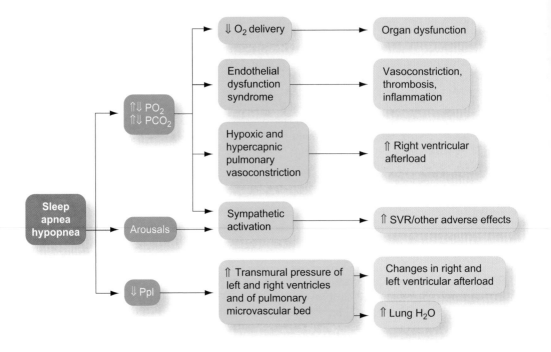

Fig. 1. Pathophysiologic consequences of sleep apnea.

blood pressure was highest during the mild hyperventilation occurring after termination of apnea (*P*<.0001).

Solin and colleagues [41] measured the overnight urinary norepinephrine (UNE) level, which is a measure of integrated overnight sympathetic activity while asleep, in 15 healthy male volunteers, 15 male OSA patients who did not have CHF, and 90 CHF patients (77 men). Compared with healthy individuals, the mean UNE level was significantly elevated in the OSA group and was even further elevated in the CHF group (13.4 plus or minus 5.6 nmol/mmol versus 19.7 plus or minus 12.3 nmol/mmol versus 32.2 plus or minus 20.2 nmol/mmol creatinine, respectively; *P*<.001). Within the CHF group, the mean UNE levels were greatest in the CHF/HCSB group, compared with the CHF/OSA group and the CHF nonapneic group (43.9 plus or minus 24.1 nmol/mmol versus 24.0 plus or minus 10.8 nmol/mmol versus 22.4 plus or minus 8.9 nmol/mmol creatinine, respectively; *P*<.001). Using a multivariate regression model, the variance of the UNE level in the CHF group was predicted, in descending order, by pulmonary capillary wedge pressure (14% variance), rapid eye movement sleep (8%), and the mean sleep pulse oximetry level (7%). The investigators concluded that overnight sympathetic activity is significantly greater in CHF patients than in OSA patients. Moreover, the hemodynamic severity of CHF contributes to the elevation of sympathetic activity in CHF

patients to a greater degree than the apnea-related hypoxemia.

An association between CSA and nocturnal ventricular arrhythmias (ie, PVCs, couplets, and ventricular tachycardia) have been well documented [11,12] and a cause-effect relationship has also been suggested. In this study by Javaheri [29], CPAP was used to treat central sleep apena in subjects with systolic heart failure. In subjects who responded to CPAP and in whom CSA was eliminated, the number of PVCs and couplets decreased significantly. The number of ventricular tachycardia also decreased but this was not as significant as the number of observations were small. In contrast, in heart failure subjects whose CSA did not respond to CPAP, the number of ventricular arrhythmias did not change significantly. In a different study [42], ventricular premature beats were found to occur 40% more frequently during the hyperpneic phase than the apneic phase of CSA (7.0 plus or minus 7.4 versus 4.9 plus or minus 5.7 ventricular premature beats per minute; *P* = .003). Ventricular premature beat frequency was also found to be higher during periods of HCSB/CSA than during periods of regular breathing, occurring either spontaneously or induced through inhalation of carbon dioxide. This increase in ventricular premature beats might contribute to the higher mortality rates reported in heart failure patients with CSA.

Atrial fibrillation is also common in CHF patients with HCSB-CSA [11,22]. It has been suggested that

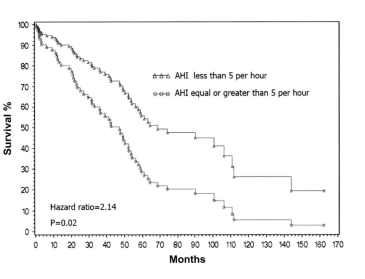

Fig. 2. Survival of patients with heart failure, with or without central sleep apnea, after accounting for all confounders. (*From* Javaheri S, Shukla R, Zeigler H, et al. Central sleep apnea, right ventricular dysfunction, and low diastolic blood pressure are predictors of mortality in systolic heart failure. J Am Coll Cardiol 2007;49:2028; with permission.)

atrial fibrillation represents a predictive factor for CSA [22] and also a risk factor for decreasing cardiac output when treating these subjects with CPAP [43].

All three factors—sympathetic activation, ventricular arrhythmia, and atrial fibrillation—along with other consequences of sleep apnea, such as hypoxemia, may act in concert and contribute to progression of heart failure. There is thus a rationale for CSA not only as a marker of the severity of CHF, but also as a risk factor for heart failure aggravation.

Impact of CSA on mortality

CSA may increase the risk of mortality in CHF [14–18]. Findley and colleagues [15] were the first to report that CSA was associated with increased mortality in patients with systolic heart failure. However, several recent studies have reported conflicting results. A major criticism in most studies is the small number of subjects, either in the CSA or in the control group. In addition, some of the studies combined cardiac transplantation with death as the primary endpoint. Most studies only reported limited variables, making it difficult to assess the effects of confounders on survival. Inclusion of patients with obstructive sleep apnea with CSA in some studies has resulted in inhomogeneity, making it difficult to interpret the results. In some studies full polysomnography was not performed.

In a recent study, Javaheri and colleagues [17] reported that central sleep apnea, independent of other factors, contributes to mortality of patients with systolic heart failure. This has been the largest and most systematic study, involving 88 subjects, 32 without CSA and 56 with CSA of various severities. The mean AHI of patients without CSA was two per hour, and was 34 per hour in those subjects

with CSA. In Cox multiple regression analysis, three factors including CSA, severity of right ventricular dysfunction, and low diastolic blood pressure, were the three independent variables predicting mortality. The median survival of patients of CSA was 45 months, compared with 90 months in those without CSA (hazard ratio = 2.14, *P* = .02) (Fig. 2).

Summary

Sleep apnea is commonly found in patients with systolic heart failure, and recent studies strongly suggest that the prevalence of central sleep apnea remains high, in spite of the use of contemporary treatment of heart failure including β-blockers. Furthermore, it has been shown that CSA may contribute to mortality of heart failure patients. However, the impact of therapy of sleep apnea on survival of heart failure patients needs to be further determined.

References

[1] Hunt SA, Abraham WT, Chin MH, et al. ACC/AHA 2005 guideline update for the diagnosis and management of chronic heart failure in the adult: a report of the American college of cardiology/American Heart Association task force on practice guidelines (Writing Committee to Update the 2001 Guidelines for the Evaluation and Management of Heart Failure): developed in collaboration with the American college of chest physicians and the international society for heart and lung transplantation: endorsed by the Heart rhythm society. Circulation 2005;112: e154–235.

[2] Jessup M, Brozena S. Heart failure. N Engl J Med 2003;348:2007–18.

[3] Ceia F, Fonseca C, Mota T, et al. Prevalence of chronic heart failure in Southwestern Europe: the EPICA study. Eur J Heart Fail 2002;4:531–9.

[4] Hoes AW, Mosterd A, Grobbee DE. An epidemic of heart failure? Recent evidence from Europe. Eur Heart J 1998;19(Suppl L):L2–9.

[5] van der Meer P, Voors AA, Lipsic E, et al. Prognostic value of plasma erythropoietin on mortality in patients with chronic heart failure. J Am Coll Cardiol 2004;44:63–7.

[6] Pocock SJ, Wang D, Pfeffer MA, et al. Predictors of mortality and morbidity in patients with chronic heart failure. Eur Heart J 2006;27:65–75.

[7] Siirila-Waris K, Lassus J, Melin J, et al. Characteristics, outcomes, and predictors of 1-year mortality in patients hospitalized for acute heart failure. Eur Heart J 2006;27:3011–7.

[8] Schaufelberger M, Swedberg K, Koster M, et al. Decreasing one-year mortality and hospitalization rates for heart failure in Sweden; Data from the Swedish Hospital Discharge Registry 1988 to 2000. Eur Heart J 2004;25:300–7.

[9] Muntwyler J, Abetel G, Gruner C, et al. One-year mortality among unselected outpatients with heart failure. Eur Heart J 2002;23:1861–6.

[10] Martinez-Selles M, Garcia Robles JA, Prieto L, et al. Systolic dysfunction is a predictor of long term mortality in men but not in women with heart failure. Eur Heart J 2003;24:2046–53.

[11] Javaheri S, Parker TJ, Liming JD, et al. Sleep apnea in 81 ambulatory male patients with stable heart failure. Types and their prevalences, consequences, and presentations. Circulation 1998;97:2154–9.

[12] Tremel F, Pepin JL, Veale D, et al. High prevalence and persistence of sleep apnoea in patients referred for acute left ventricular failure and medically treated over 2 months. Eur Heart J 1999;20:1201–9.

[13] Sin DD, Fitzgerald F, Parker JD, et al. Risk factors for central and obstructive sleep apnea in 450 men and women with congestive heart failure. Am J Respir Crit Care Med 1999;160:1101–6.

[14] Lofaso F, Verschueren P, Rande JL, et al. Prevalence of sleep-disordered breathing in patients on a heart transplant waiting list. Chest 1994;106:1689–94.

[15] Findley LJ, Zwillich CW, Ancoli-Israel S, et al. Cheyne-Stokes breathing during sleep in patients with left ventricular heart failure. South Med J 1985;78:11–5.

[16] Lanfranchi PA, Braghiroli A, Bosimini E, et al. Prognostic value of nocturnal Cheyne-stokes respiration in chronic heart failure. Circulation 1999;99:1435–40.

[17] Javaheri S, Shukla R, Zeigler H, et al. Central sleep apnea, right ventricular dysfunction, and low diastolic blood pressure are predictors of mortality in systolic heart failure. J Am Coll Cardiol 2007;49:2028–34.

[18] Roebuck T, Solin P, Kaye DM, et al. Increased long-term mortality in heart failure due to sleep apnoea is not yet proven. Eur Respir J 2004;23:735–40.

[19] Andreas S, Hagenah G, Moller C, et al. Cheyne-Stokes respiration and prognosis in congestive heart failure. Am J Cardiol 1996;78:1260–4.

[20] Javaheri S, Parker TJ, Wexler L, et al. Occult sleep-disordered breathing in stable congestive heart failure. Ann Intern Med 1995;122:487–92.

[21] Lanfranchi PA, Somers VK, Braghiroli A, et al. Central sleep apnea in left ventricular dysfunction: prevalence and implications for arrhythmic risk. Circulation 2003;107:727–32.

[22] Javaheri S. Sleep disorders in systolic heart failure: a prospective study of 100 male patients. The final report. Int J Cardiol 2006;106:21–8.

[23] Bradley TD, Logan AG, Kimoff RJ, et al. Continuous positive airway pressure for central sleep apnea and heart failure. N Engl J Med 2005;353:2025–33.

[24] Ferrier K, Campbell A, Yee B, et al. Sleep-disordered breathing occurs frequently in stable outpatients with congestive heart failure. Chest 2005;128:2116–22.

[25] Schulz R, Blau A, Borgel J, et al. Sleep apnoea in heart failure. Eur Respir J 2007;29(6):1201–5.

[26] Oldenburg O, Lamp B, Faber L, et al. Sleep-disordered breathing in patients with symptomatic heart failure A contemporary study of prevalence in and characteristics of 700 patients. Eur J Heart Failure 2007;9:251–7.

[27] Vazir A, Hastings PC, Dayer M, et al. A high prevalence of sleep disordered breathing in men with mild symptomatic chronic heart failure due to left ventricular systolic dysfunction. Eur J Heart Failure 2007;9:243–50.

[28] Zhao Z, Sullivan C, Liu Z, et al. Prevalence and clinical characteristics of sleep apnea in Chinese patients with heart failure. Int J Cardiol 2007;118:122–3.

[29] Javaheri S. Effects of continuous positive airway pressure on sleep apnea and ventricular irritability in patients with heart failure. Circulation 2000;101:392–7.

[30] Garrigue S, Pepin JL, Defaye P, et al. High prevalence of sleep apnea syndrome in patients with long-term pacing: the European Multicenter Polysomnographic Study. Circulation 2007;115(13):1703–9.

[31] Feldman AM, de Lissovoy G, Bristow MR, et al. Cost effectiveness of cardiac resynchronization therapy in the comparison of medical therapy, pacing, and defibrillation in heart failure (COMPANION) trial. J Am Coll Cardiol 2005;46:2311–21.

[32] Lindenfeld J, Feldman AM, Saxon L, et al. Effects of cardiac resynchronization therapy with or without a defibrillator on survival and hospitalizations in patients with New York Heart Association class IV heart failure. Circulation 2007;115:204–12.

[33] Sinha AM, Skobel EC, Breithardt OA, et al. Cardiac resynchronization therapy improves central

sleep apnea and Cheyne-Stokes respiration in patients with chronic heart failure. J Am Coll Cardiol 2004;44:68–71.

[34] Oldenburg O, Faber L, Vogt J, et al. Influence of cardiac resynchronisation therapy on different types of sleep disordered breathing. Eur J Heart Fail 2007;9(8):820–6.

[35] Javaheri S. Sleep-related breathing disorders in heart failure. In: Heart failure, A companion to Braunwald's Heart Disease. Douglas L. Mann, editor. WB Saunders, Philadelphia, 2004; 471–87.

[36] Wuyam B, Pepin JL, Tremel F, et al. Pathophysiology of central sleep apnea syndrome. Sleep 2000;23(Suppl 4):S213–9.

[37] Pepin JL, Chouri-Pontarollo N, Tamisier R, et al. Cheyne-Stokes respiration with central sleep apnoea in chronic heart failure: proposals for a diagnostic and therapeutic strategy. Sleep Med Rev 2006;10:33–47.

[38] Javaheri S. Heart failure. In: Principles and practices of sleep medicine, 4/e; Kryger MH, Roth T, Dement WC, editors; WB Saunders, Philadelphia, 2005;1208–17.

[39] Javaheri S, Wexler L. Prevalence and treatment of breathing disorders during sleep in heart failure patients. Curr Treat Options Cardiovasc Med 2005;7:295–305.

[40] van de Borne P, Oren R, Abouassaly C, et al. Effect of Cheyne-Stokes respiration on muscle sympathetic nerve activity in severe congestive heart failure secondary to ischemic or idiopathic dilated cardiomyopathy. Am J Cardiol 1998;81:432–6.

[41] Solin P, Kaye DM, Little PJ, et al. Impact of sleep apnea on sympathetic nervous system activity in heart failure. Chest 2003;123:1119–26.

[42] Leung RS, Diep TM, Bowman ME, et al. Provocation of ventricular ectopy by Cheyne-Stokes respiration in patients with heart failure. Sleep 2004;27:1337–43.

[43] Liston R, Deegan PC, McCreery C, et al. Haemodynamic effects of nasal continuous positive airway pressure in severe congestive heart failure. Eur Respir J 1995;8:430–5.

ELSEVIER
SAUNDERS

SLEEP
MEDICINE
CLINICS

Sleep Med Clin 2 (2007) 623–630

Mechanisms of Sleep Apnea and Periodic Breathing in Systolic Heart Failure

Shahrokh Javaheri, MD[a],*, J.A. Dempsey, PhD[b]

Central sleep apnea (CSA) is caused by temporary failure in breathing rhythm generation resulting in the loss of inspiratory effort. During CSA, there is no medullary inspiratory neural output to the diaphragm and other inspiratory thoracic pump muscles. Polygraphically, CSA is characterized by the absence of thoracoabdominal excursions and naso-oral airflow. In contrast, an obstructive sleep apnea (OSA) is caused by relaxation of the oropharyngeal muscles and occlusion of the upper airway in the presence of continual rhythmic contractions of inspiratory thoracic pump muscles. Polygraphically, OSA is characterized by the absence of naso-oral airflow despite thoracoabdominal excursions.

There are many causes of CSA [1], with systolic heart failure being the most common cause. Both OSA and CSA commonly occur in patients with systolic heart failure, however, and frequently simultaneously in the same patient. Appreciating this phenomenon, for pathophysiologic and therapeutic reasons the authors have classified patients into predominantly OSA or CSA [2–4]. This categorization was based on arbitrary polysomnographic findings. It must be emphasized, however, that in systolic heart failure both OSA and CSA occur in the background of Hunter-Cheyne-Stokes breathing, a pattern of breathing unique to heart failure.

This article reviews the mechanisms of CSA, OSA, and periodic breathing in systolic heart failure.

Control of breathing

Three distinct control systems influence breathing: (1) the automatic-metabolic system; (2) state of wakefulness (versus sleep); and (3) behavioral control of breathing [5]. The latter is best exemplified by

The research studies of the authors were supported in part by a grant from NHLBI (J.A.D.) and the Veterans' Administration (S.J. and J.A.D.).
[a] Sleepcare Diagnostics, 4780 Socialville-Fosters Rd., Mason, OH 45040, USA
[b] John Rankin Laboratory of Pulmonary Medicine, University of Wisconsin, Madison, Wisconsin, USA
* Corresponding author. Sleepcare Diagnostics, 4780 Socialville-Fosters Rd., Mason, OH 45040.
E-mail address: javaheri@snorenomore.com (S. Javaheri).

doi:10.1016/j.jsmc.2007.07.005

the circumstances when the respiratory system is used for functions, such as talking, swallowing, or laughing, and is not discussed further in this article.

The automatic-metabolic system controls both the automatic act of breathing and the coupling of ventilation to the metabolic rate. The various components of this system include a central pacemaker, presumably located in the pre-Botzinger complex; the pontomedullary respiratory centers (the dorsal and ventral respiratory groups); and a number of receptors. The main receptors include the chemoreceptors (the peripheral arterial chemoreceptors in the carotid bodies located between internal and external carotid arteries, and the medullary central chemoreceptors located in the medulla oblongata) and a number of intrathoracic receptors, such as J receptors. The peripheral and the central chemoreceptors are involved in the chemoreflex control of breathing, a negative feedback system; their activity is regulated by P_{O_2} and P_{CO_2}/$H+$ [5]. The J receptors are stimulated by the pathologic processes in the lung, and by the vagus nerve have afferent input to the respiratory centers. The end result of stimulation of J receptors is tachypnea, as seen in pulmonary congestion and edema.

In brief, the automatic-metabolic control system is responsible for the act of breathing (automatic) and also maintaining arterial P_{O_2} and $[H^+]$ relatively constant by coupling alveolar ventilation to metabolic rate (metabolic control). Any disturbance in breathing that changes P_{O_2}, or $[H^+]$ alters the activity of the chemoreceptors and consequently ventilation is changed in such a way that the magnitude of the initial disturbance is minimized (a negative feedback system). Under normal circumstances, P_{CO_2} is the most important variable controlling breathing, because any small change in P_{CO_2} affects ventilation. This P_{CO_2} effect is critically important in maintaining rhythmic breathing during sleep when ventilation is strictly regulated by the metabolic control system (see later).

The state of wakefulness has a major influence on breathing (wakefulness drive) and this is mediated through suprapontine neural input to the brainstem respiratory pattern generator. The suprapontine neural activity is in turn regulated by the afferent excitatory input from the ascending reticular activating system, part of the brain arousal system located in the brainstem. The arousal system consists of multiple neural structures, rich in various neurotransmitters. Some of these structures are the locus ceruleus (norepinephrine); the dorsal raphe (serotonin); the tuberomammillary nucleus (histamine); and the laterodorsal and pedunculopontine tegmental nuclei (acetylcholine). These neural structures are active during wakefulness and their activity decreases with onset of non–rapid eye movement (REM) sleep. As a result, there is loss of suprapontine neural input to the respiratory centers and loss of wakefulness drive to breathe. Consequently, during non-REM sleep, breathing comes under the metabolic control system (the negative feedback system). The loss of wakefulness drive for breathing is critical, because the metabolic control system is sensitive to small changes in P_{CO_2}, and sleep unmasks a very P_{CO_2}-sensitive apneic threshold. This sets the stage for development of central apneas during sleep.

Concept of apneic threshold and ventilatory response to CO_2 below eupnea during sleep

The mechanisms involved in the genesis of central apnea relate specifically to the state of sleep and removal of wakefulness drive on breathing. This unmasks the apneic threshold P_{CO_2} [6–9], a P_{CO_2} level below which rhythmic breathing ceases resulting in CSA.

Normally with onset of sleep, ventilation decreases and P_{CO_2} rises by a few millimeters of mercury. If the spontaneous prevailing P_{CO_2}, referred to as the "eupneic P_{CO_2}," decreases below the apneic threshold P_{CO_2}, breathing ceases. Apneic threshold P_{CO_2} is numerically close to awake P_{CO_2} [10]; the small rise in eupneic P_{CO_2} with sleep onset is critically important to maintain breathing. Inability to increase eupneic P_{CO_2} with sleep onset is critical to development of central sleep in congestive heart failure. When eupneic P_{CO_2} decreases below apneic threshold P_{CO_2}, CSA occurs. As a result of CSA, P_{CO_2} rises and after it exceeds the apneic threshold P_{CO_2}, breathing resumes. The difference between two P_{CO_2} set points, the eupneic P_{CO_2} minus the P_{CO_2} at the apneic threshold (P_{CO_2} reserve), is a critical factor for development of CSA (Figs. 1 and 2) [11,12]. The smaller this difference, the greater the likelihood of occurrence of CSA. This is because small increases in ventilation could lower the eupneic P_{CO_2} below the apneic threshold (see Fig. 1). When eupneic P_{CO_2} is far above the apneic threshold P_{CO_2}, however, large ventilatory changes are necessary to lower the P_{CO_2} below the apneic threshold, decreasing the likelihood of developing central apnea. In the genesis of CSA, the difference between the two P_{CO_2} set points rather that the actual value of the eupneic P_{CO_2} is critical. In contrast to the general belief, a low P_{CO_2} by itself is protective against development of CSA. This was revealed in a polysomnographic study of hypocapnic patients with cirrhosis of the liver, which showed absence of CSA in this population [13]. This phenomenon is related to the alveolar-ventilation equation and where P_{CO_2} is in relation to ventilation on the isometabolic hyperbola. Accordingly,

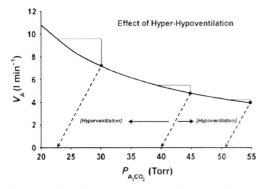

Fig. 1. Relationship of alveolar Pco₂ (Paco₂) with alveolar ventilation (VA). The intersection of the dotted lines with the X access shows apneic threshold. As noted, when Paco₂ decreases (metabolic acidosis) the difference between the eucapnic Paco₂ and apneic threshold Pco₂ increases making it less likely to develop central sleep apnea. The opposite is true in the face of metabolic alkalosis when compared with normal ventilation (control).

when steady-state hyperventilation is present and Pco₂ is low, if the sensitivity to CO₂ below eupnea is unchanged, the Pco₂ reserve increases (proportional to the degree of hyperventilation), making it less likely to develop central apnea during sleep (see Fig. 1) [11,12]. This, for example, occurs in metabolic acidosis induced by acetazolamide (see Fig. 1) [9], which is used to treat CSA in congestive heart failure [14]. In contrast, when CO₂ sensitivity

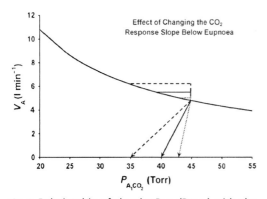

Fig. 2. Relationship of alveolar Pco₂ (Paco₂) with alveolar ventilation (VA) and three conditions of control (*solid arrow*), congestive heart failure with central sleep apnea, and also hypoxia (*broken arrow*), and hyperventilation with metabolic acidosis (*dotted arrow*). As noted, both hypoxia and congestive heart failure with central sleep apnea increase the slope of the ventilatory response below eupnoea increasing the likelihood of developing central sleep apnea. In contrast, hyperventilation and metabolic acidosis decrease the slope of the ventilatory response below eupnoea and the likelihood of developing central sleep apnea.

below eupnea is increased, the Pco₂ reserve decreases, and this increases the likelihood of developing central apnea during sleep (see Fig. 2) [15]. This occurs experimentally with dopamine infusion [11,12], and in some patients with systolic heart failure who develop central apnea during sleep (see Fig. 2) [11,12,15].

Central apnea is precipitated by sleep, because of unmasking of the apneic threshold. Like OSA, CSA does not occur during wakefulness, although at times during polysomnography it is observed that some patients develop CSA or OSA when alpha wave is predominant and the epoch may be scored awake. With careful observation of electroencephalogram, however, slowing of brain waves is observed when either CSA or OSA occurs.

With this background, the mechanisms of CSA and periodic breathing are discussed, followed by mechanisms of OSA in systolic heart failure.

Mechanisms of central sleep apnea and periodic breathing in systolic heart failure

Hunter-Cheyne-Stokes breathing is a form of periodic breathing with a distinctive feature characterized by long cycle of ventilatory instability. Prolonged waxing and waning changes in tidal volume commonly with an intervening central apnea or hypopnea are characteristic features of this form of periodic breathing. The prolonged cycle of ventilatory instability reflects the prolonged arterial circulation time, a pathologic feature of systolic heart failure. This prolonged cycle of ventilatory instability distinguishes this form of periodic breathing from other phenotypes of periodic breathing [1], such as the idiopathic form of CSA, opioid-induced CSA, and the periodic breathing caused by hypoxia at high altitude; in all of these the cycle length is short, and there is no crescendo out of the apnea (cluster-type breathing pattern).

Next, a distinction is made between the mechanisms of CSA and the mechanisms mediating periodic breathing. This distinction is in part for simplicity because the mechanisms overlap. This distinction is important because genesis of CSA has to do primarily with the removal of wakefulness drive and the unmasking of the apneic threshold with sleep onset. This means that CSA, like OSA, is a sleep-state specific. In contrast, the mechanisms mediating periodic breathing have to do with the pathologic processes of heart failure (eg, increased arterial circulation time noted previously) [16]. Such pathologic processes of heart failure are not state-specific. It is not surprising that in patients with systolic heart failure periodic breathing may be observed during wakefulness and even during exercise [17]. Sleep also has a profound effect, however, on periodic breathing. This is because the pathophysiologic processes of heart failure mediating periodic breathing are further augmented during sleep (discussed later). As a result, many patients with heart failure have periodic breathing only during sleep and not while they are awake [18].

Central sleep apnea in systolic heart failure

Normally, with the onset of sleep, respiratory rate and tidal volume decrease and Pco_2 increases. This keeps the eupneic Pco_2 above the apneic threshold Pco_2, maintaining rhythmic breathing while asleep. In some patients with heart failure, however, the prevailing awake Pco_2 does not rise during sleep [15,16]. Because of the proximity of the eupneic Pco_2 to the exposed apneic threshold, the likelihood of developing CSA increases. Furthermore, in heart failure patients with CSA, hypocapneic CO_2 sensitivity is increased resulting in further predisposition to CSA (see Fig. 2) [15].

The reason for the lack of normally observed sleep-induced rise in Pco_2 in some patients with heart failure is not clear. One possibility could be the lack of normally observed sleep-induced decrease in ventilation, which could be difficult to measure because the changes are small. It is assumed that in those heart failure patients with most severe left ventricular diastolic dysfunction (which invariably accompanies systolic dysfunction) pulmonary capillary pressure rises further when venous return increases in supine position. This results in a small increase in respiratory rate and ventilation (caused by stimulation of receptors in cardiopulmonary systems [eg, J receptors]), preventing the normally observed rise in Pco_2. Because the increase in respiratory rate is small, the increment may only be detected (to become statistically significant) if a large number of patients are studied. Measurements of central hemodynamics and $Paco_2$ in sitting position while awake and in supine position while asleep may be necessary to provide the evidence. In this context, in naturally sleeping dogs, acute elevation in left atrial pressure (and the resultant increase in pulmonary capillary pressure) decreases Pco_2 and increases CO_2 sensitivity below eupnoea, increasing the propensity for development of CSA [19]. The mechanism of a reduced Pco_2 reserve in heart failure is not known. One potential mechanism could be reduced cerebrovascular response to hypocapnia in patients with heart failure and CSA when compared with heart failure patients without CSA [20]. Independent of the mechanism, the result of this study [19] also explains the observation from studies [21–23] that have shown that subjects with heart failure and

low $Paco_2$ have a high probability of developing central apnea during sleep. In one study, the predictive value of a low awake $Paco_2$ for development of CSA was about 80% [23]. The result of this study [19] is also consistent with the notion that the severity of the left ventricular diastolic dysfunction, reflected in progressively increasing pulmonary capillary pressure, correlates with $Paco_2$ [24].

Heart failure patients with hypocapnia have left ventricular diastolic dysfunction and a high pulmonary capillary pressure. Because of diastolic dysfunction, pulmonary capillary pressure should further increase during supine position as venous return increases; this should result in a decrease in Pco_2 reserve increasing the propensity to develop CSA during sleep.

It is emphasized that although a low awake $Paco_2$ is highly predictive of CSA [23], it is not a prerequisite. Most patients with heart failure and CSA have normal awake $Paco_2$ [23,25]. What is important is the proximity of the $Paco_2$ to the apneic threshold and the increased chemosensitivity below eupnoea.

Two other implications of the Pco_2 reserve relate to the observation that CSA is less common in REM than non-REM sleep, and also in women (than in men) with heart failure. Regarding REM sleep, from a cerebral neurophysiologic point of view, this sleep state resembles wakefulness. For example, in contrast to non-REM sleep and similar to wakefulness, cerebral blood flow and glucose use are increased; the laterodorsal and pedunculopontine tegmental nuclei, part of the reticular activating system, are active in REM sleep; and also the brain waves to some extent resemble wakefulness. This may explain the observations of Xi and colleagues [26] that Pco_2 reserve increases during phasic REM sleep making it more difficult to develop CSA.

Regarding gender, although definitive studies have not been performed, combining the results of several studies (reviewed in [2]) shows that prevalence of CSA is lower in female than male patients with systolic heart failure. The risk of CSA increases after menopause, however, being six times higher in those 60 years or older than those less than 60 years [27]. Premenopausal women have a lower apneic threshold than men [28], and this may be in part the reason for a lower prevalence of CSA in premenopausal women than in men with heart failure. The lower apneic threshold in women than in men could be mediated by the balance between the level of female [28] and male hormones [29].

Mechanisms of periodic breathing in systolic heart failure

In heart failure, central apneas occur in the background of periodic breathing. This unique pattern of breathing is characterized by long cresendo-decresendo arms. The mechanisms underlying this breathing pattern are to some extent distinct from those mediating development of central apnea, although some of the mechanisms overlap.

Metabolic control of breathing is a negative feedback system [1,5]. Mathematical and experimental models [30,31] of the negative feedback system controlling breathing predict that increased arterial circulation time (increased mixing gain), which delays the transfer of information regarding changes in P_{O_2} and P_{CO_2} from pulmonary capillary blood to the chemoreceptors, increased sensitivity of the chemoreceptors (increased controller gain), and increased plant gain (a large change in P_{aCO_2} for a small change in ventilation) collectively increase the likelihood of periodic breathing. These three factors are present in some patients with systolic heart failure. It is not surprising that heart failure is so conducive to development of period breathing. First, in systolic heart failure, effective arterial circulation time (mixing gain) is increased for a variety of reasons, such as pulmonary congestion, left atrial and ventricular enlargement, and diminished stroke volume. Second, a low functional residual capacity increases the plant gain, although this could be opposed if steady-state P_{CO_2} is low. Functional residual capacity could be decreased because of pleural effusion, cardiomegaly, pulmonary congestion, or edema. Third, in some patients with heart failure, hypercapnic ventilatory response above eupnea

(controller gain) is increased [32]. The latter has been shown to be another distinguishing feature between those heart failure patients with or without periodic breathing and central apnea during sleep. In such individuals with increased sensitivity to carbon dioxide, the chemoreceptors elicit a transitory large ventilatory response whenever the partial pressure of carbon dioxide rises (this may happen during an arousal). The consequent intense hyperventilation, by driving the P_{CO_2} below the apneic threshold, results in CSA. Because of CSA, P_{CO_2} rises. The cycles of hyperventilation and hypoventilation (periodic breathing and CSA) are maintained. Meanwhile, because of a long circulation time, hyperventilation continues longer than if circulation time was normal and short.

The increased controller gain above eupnea is particularly important during arousals when upper airway resistance decreases, and the sleeping P_{CO_2} becomes hypercapnic for the aroused brain. These two arousal-related changes result in intense hyperventilation. When sleep resumes, the P_{CO_2} is hypocapnic for the chemoreceptors resulting in CSA. In a study of patients with systolic heart failure, CO_2 chemosensitivity above eupnea directly correlated with central apnea index [32].

In heart failure, the combination of increased controller gain, mixing gain, and plant gain destabilizes breathing both during wakefulness and sleep. Sleep (and also supine position), however,

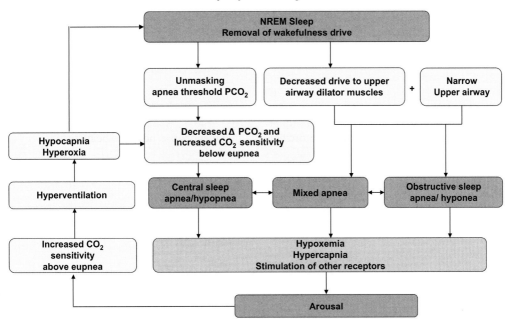

Fig. 3. Schematic depiction of the overlapping mechanisms mediating central, mixed, and obstructive sleep apnea in systolic heart failure.

promotes periodic breathing further. In supine position and during sleep, cardiac output decreases (further prolonging arterial circulation time), and both functional residual capacity and metabolic rate decrease enhancing the plant gain. All these alterations increase the likelihood of developing periodic breathing during sleep. In addition, in supine position, venous return increases resulting in an increase in pulmonary capillary wedge pressure and a decrease in Pco_2 reserve during sleep.

Next, some treatment options as they relate to the mechanisms of CSA are mentioned. In naturally sleeping dogs, Nakayama and colleagues [9] showed that acetazolamide decreased the plant gain (with no change in controller gain), increasing the Pco_2 reserve and decreasing the propensity to develop CSA (see Fig. 1). In a double-blind, placebo-controlled study [14] of 12 patients with systolic heart failure, acetazolamide significantly decreased the number of central apneas. This occurred despite acetazolamide-induced lowering of $Paco_2$ (caused by metabolic acidosis). The results of this study [14] are consistent with the principle that a low $Paco_2$ per se is protective against development of CSA, a notion also consistent with absence of CSA in hypocapnic patients with cirrhosis [13].

Several studies have shown that administration of supplemental oxygen improves CSA [33]. The mechanisms include decreasing hypercapnic ventilatory drive above eupnea and perhaps below eupnea. Although the latter has not been tested directly, it has been shown that hypoxemia increases the CO_2 chemosensitivity below eupnea and decreases Pco_2 reserve (see Fig. 2). Administration of O_2 also increases $Paco_2$, which may increase Pco_2 reserve, but at the same time should also increase the plant gain. Finally, both addition of dead space [34,35] and CO_2 inhalation [36–39] also decrease the number of central apneas. These modalities increase ventilation decreasing the plant gain; meanwhile, breathing with an elevated inspired CO_2 always prevents Pco_2 from falling, regardless of the level of ventilation, transient or steady state. The lack of fall in Pco_2 eliminates ventilatory inhibition. Inhalation of CO_2, which increases $Paco_2$ by about 2 to 3 mm Hg, may increase arousals and sympathetic actually [35,38] and is not an appropriate therapeutic modality for treatment of CSA in patients with systolic heart failure.

Mechanisms of obstructive sleep apnea and systolic heart failure

In patients with systolic heart failure, it is common to see both OSA and CSA in the same patient. For this reason, the authors have categorized the polysomnograms into predominantly OSA or predominantly CSA [18,40,41]. The frequent occurrence of OSA with CSA in patients with systolic heart failure is to a large extent in contrast to patients with OSA and without heart failure. There are reasons for simultaneous occurrence of OSA and CSA in patients with systolic heart failure (Fig. 3). Because of increased circulation time, patients with systolic heart failure are prone to periodic breathing, and obstructive disordered breathing occurs at the nadir of periodic breathing. In one study [42] in which the authors placed an esophageal balloon in sleeping patients with heart failure, it was noticed that episodes of obstruction occurred at the end of the central apneas (events normally classified as mixed apnea) in almost one third of the patients. This is in line with the concept that the neural output to the muscles of the upper airway is particularly reduced during nadir of the ventilation and the direct bronchoscopic observation [43] of upper airway narrowing and closure during central apneas.

Upper airway closure is particularly apt to occur in heart failure patients with anatomically narrow upper airway. In studies in which polysomnograms were scored blindly and then matched with demographics of the patients [40,41], it was found that those polysomnograms classified as predominant OSA belonged to heart failure patients who were obese and had a high prevalence of habitual snoring. This is consistent with findings during hypoxia-induced periodic breathing when upper airway occlusion occurs at the nadir ventilation only in those subjects with increased upper airway resistance and collapsible airway [44].

Summary

Periodic breathing and CSA are common in patients with systolic heart failure. The mechanisms of CSA are complex. Recent studies have demonstrated that those patients with systolic heart failure who have increased CO_2 chemosensitivity below and above eupnea are prone to develop central apnea during sleep. OSA also occurs frequently in patients with heart failure, particularly in those with obesity who presumably have alterations in the mechanical properties of the upper airway.

References

[1] Javaheri S. Central sleep apnea in sleep: a comprehensive handbook. In: Lee-Chiong TL, editor. New Jersey: Wiley-Liss; 2006. p. 246–62.
[2] Javaheri S. Heart failure. In: Kryger MH, Roth T, Dement WC, editors. Principles and practices of sleep medicine. 4th edition. Philadelphia: WB Saunders Company; 2005.

[3] Javaheri S. Central sleep apnea in congestive heart failure: prevalence, mechanisms, impacts and therapeutic options. Semin Respir Crit Care Med 2005;26(1):44–55.

[4] Javaheri S. Sleep-related breathing disorders in heart failure. In: Mann DL, editor. Heart failure, a companion to Braunwald's heart disease. Philadelphia: WB Saunders; 2004. p. 471–87.

[5] Javaheri S. Determinants of carbon dioxide tension. In: Gennari FJ, Adrogue HJ, Galla JH, et al, editors. Acid-base disorders. Boca Raton (FL): Taylor & Francis Group; 2005. p. 47–77.

[6] Dempsey JA, Skatrud JB. Fundamental effects of sleep state on breathing. Curr Pulmonol 1988; 9:267–304.

[7] Skatrud JB, Dempsey JA. Interaction of sleep state and chemical stimuli in sustaining rhythmic ventilation. J Appl Physiol 1983;55:813–22.

[8] Dempsey JA, Skatrud JB. A sleep-induced apneic threshold and its consequences. Am Rev Respir Dis 1986;133:1163–70.

[9] Nakayama H, Smith CA, Rodman JR, et al. Effect of ventilatory drive on CO_2 sensitivity below eupnea during sleep. AM J Critical Care Med 2002;165:1251–8.

[10] Thomson S, Morrell M, Cordingley J, et al. Ventilation is unstable during drowsiness before sleep onset. J Appl Physiol 2005;99:2036–44.

[11] Dempsey J, Smith C, Przybylowski T, et al. The ventilatory responsiveness to CO_2 below eupnoea as a determinant of ventilatory stability in sleep. J Physio 2004;560:1–11.

[12] Dempsey J. Crossing the apnoeic threshold: causes and consequences. Exp Physiol 2004; 90(1):13–24.

[13] Javaheri S, Almoosa K, Saleh K, et al. Hypocapnia is not a predictor of central sleep apnea in patients with cirrhosis. Am J Respir Crit Care Med 2005;171:908–11.

[14] Javaheri S. Acetazolamide improves central sleep apnea in heart failure: a double-blind prospective study. Am J Respir Crit Care Med 2006;173:234–7.

[15] Xie A, Skatrud JB, Puleo DS, et al. Apnea-hypopnea threshold for CO_2 in patients with congestive heart failure. Am J Respir Crit Care Med 2002;165:1245–50.

[16] Hall MJ, Xie A, Rutherford R, et al. Cycle length of periodic breathing in patients with and without heart failure. Am J Respir Crit Care Med 1996;154:376–81.

[17] Ponikowski P, Anker S, Chua T, et al. Oscillatory breathing patterns during wakefulness in patients with chronic heart failure. Circulation 1999;100:2418–24.

[18] Javaheri S, Parker TJ, Wexler L, et al. Occult sleep-disordered breathing in stable congestive heart failure. Ann Intern Med 1995;122:487–92 [Erratum, Ann Intern Med 1995;123:77].

[19] Chenuel B, Smith C, Skatrud J, et al. Increased propensity for apnea in response to acute elevations in left atrial pressure during sleep in the dog. J Appl Physiol 2006;101:76–83.

[20] Xie A, Skatrud J, Khayat R, et al. Cerebrovascular response to carbon dioxide in patients with congestive heart failure. Am J Respir Crit Care Med 2005;172:371–8.

[21] Hanly P, Zuberi N, Gray R. Pathogenesis of Cheyne-Stokes respiration in patients with congestive heart failure: relationship to arterial PCO_2. Chest 1993;104:1079–84.

[22] Naughton M, Bernard D, Tam A, et al. Role of hyperventilation in the pathogenesis of central sleep apneas in patients with congestive heart failure. Am Rev Respir Dis 1993;148:330–8.

[23] Javaheri S, Corbett WS. Association of low $Paco_2$ with central sleep apnea and ventricular arrhythmias in ambulatory patients with stable heart failure. Ann Intern Med 1998;128:204–7.

[24] Solin P, Bergin P, Richardson M, et al. Influence of pulmonary capillary wedge pressure on central apnea in heart failure. Circulation 1999;99:1574–9.

[25] Javaheri S. Central sleep apnea and heart failure [Letter to the editor]. Circulation 2000;342:293–4.

[26] Xi A, Lin J, Smith CA, et al. Effects of rapid eye movement sleep on the apneic threshold in dogs. J Appl Physiol 1993;75:1129–39.

[27] Sin DD, Fitzgerald F, Parker JD, et al. Risk factors for central and obstructive sleep apnea in 450 men and women with congestive heart failure. Am J Respir Crit Care Med 1999;160:1101–6.

[28] Zhou XS, Shahabuddin S, Zahn BR, et al. Effect of gender on the development of hypocapnic apnea/hypopnea during NREM sleep. J Appl Physiol 2000;89:192–9.

[29] Zhou XS, Rowley JA, Demirovic F, et al. Effect of testosterone on the apnea threshold in women during NREM sleep. J Appl Physiol 2003;94:101–7.

[30] Cherniack NS, Longobardo GS. Cheyne-stokes breathing: an instability in physiologic control. N Engl J Med 1973;288:952–7.

[31] Khoo MCK, Kronauer RE, Strohl KP, et al. Factors inducing periodic breathing in humans: a general model. J Appl Physiol 1982;53:644–59.

[32] Javaheri S. A mechanism of central sleep apnea in patients with heart failure. N Engl J Med 1999;341:949–54.

[33] Javaheri S. Pembrey's dream: time has come for a long-term trial of nocturnal supplemental nasal oxygen to treat central sleep apnea in congestive heart failure. Chest 2003;123:322–5.

[34] Khayat R, Xie A, Patel A, et al. Cardiorespiratory effects of added dead space in patients with heart failure and central sleep apnea. Chest 2003;123:1551–60.

[35] Szollosi I, O'Driscoll DM, Dayer MJ, et al. Adaptive servo-ventilation and deadspace: effects of central sleep apnoea. J Sleep Res 2006;15:199–205.

[36] Lorenzi-Filho G, Rankin F, Bies I, et al. Effects of inhaled carbon dioxide and oxygen on

Cheyne-Stokes respiration in patients with heart failure. Am J Respir Crit Care Med 1999;159:1490–8.

[37] Szollosi I, Jones M, Morrell M, et al. Effects of CO_2 inhalation on central sleep apnea and arousals from sleep. Respiration 2004;71:493–8.

[38] Andreas S, Weidel K, Hagenah G, et al. Treatment of Cheyne-Stokes respiration with nasal oxygen and carbon dioxide. Eur Respir J 1998;12:414–9.

[39] Steens R, Millar W, Xiaoling S, et al. Effects of inhaled 3% CO_2 on Cheyne-Stokes respiration in congestive heart failure. Sleep 1994;17:61–9.

[40] Javaheri S, Parker TJ, Liming JD, et al. Sleep apnea in 81 ambulatory male patients with stable heart failure: types and their prevalences, consequences, and presentations. Circulation 1998;97:2154–9.

[41] Javaheri S. Sleep disorders in 100 male patients with systolic heart failure: a prospective study. Int J Cardiol, in press.

[42] Dowdell WT, Javaheri S, McGinnis W. Cheyene-Stokes respiration presenting as sleep apnea syndrome: clinical and polysomnographic features. Am Rev Respir Dis 1990;141:871–9.

[43] Badr S, Toiber F, Skatrud J, et al. Pharyngeal narrowing/occlution during central sleep apnea. J Appl Physiol 1995;78(5):1806–915.

[44] Xi A, Skatrud J, Dempsey J. Effect of hypoxia on the hypopnoeic and apnoeic threshold for CO_2 in sleeping humans. J Physiol 2001;535(1):269–78.

ELSEVIER
SAUNDERS

SLEEP
MEDICINE
CLINICS

Sleep Med Clin 2 (2007) 631–638

Treatment of Sleep Apnea in Heart Failure

W. De Backer, MD[a],*, Shahrokh Javaheri, MD[b]

- Treatment of obstructive sleep apnea
- Treatment of central sleep apnea
  Optimization of cardiopulmonary
      function
  Cardiac transplantation

Positive airway pressure devices
Cardiac pacemakers
Medications
- Summary
- References

As emphasized elsewhere in this issue of *The Clinics*, both obstructive and central sleep apnea (OSA and CSA, respectively) are prevalent in systolic heart failure [1–3]. Depending on the predominant form of sleep apnea, there are different therapeutic options for obstructive and central sleep apnea (Box 1, Fig. 1) [4–8].

Treatment of obstructive sleep apnea

Treatment of OSA in heart failure is similar to that in the absence of heart failure, though there are some differences (see Box 1).

Optimal treatment of heart failure by improving periodic breathing may decrease the likelihood of developing upper airway occlusion, which commonly occurs at the nadir of the ventilatory cycle. Furthermore, because elevated right atrial and central venous pressure may result in pharyngeal congestion and edema, therapeutic measures to decrease venous pressure [9] and increase upper airway size is advisable.

The authors also recommend that obese heart failure patients with OSA be advised to lose weight. Obesity is associated with heart failure and

increased incidence of cardiovascular death [10,11]. In the general population, weight loss improves obstructive sleep apnea, and this should also apply to patients with heart failure with obstructive sleep apnea and obesity [2,3].

Patients should also be advised to avoid use of benzodiazepines and alcoholic beverages. These chemicals result in relaxation of the muscles of upper airway and may promote upper airway occlusion. Further, by impairing arousal system, alcohol and benzodiazepines may prolong apneas. The authors also advise avoiding sildenafil. A double blind, placebo controlled study [12] showed that a 50-mg tablet of sildenafil, administered before bedtime, resulted in significant increase in apnea-hypopnea index, from 32 to 48 per hour, and worsening of arterial oxyhemoglobin desaturation. Care should be particularly exercised in patients with primary pulmonary hypertension in whom sildenafil may be used as a pulmonary vasodilator. Such patients may suffer from sleep apnea, which could be worsened by administration of sildenafil.

Nasal positive air pressure devices, such as a continuous positive air pressure (CPAP) device, have been successfully used to treat obstructive sleep

[a] Department of Pulmonary Medicine, University Hospital Antwerp, Wilrijkstraat 10 B-2650, Edegem, Belgium
[b] Sleepcare Diagnostics, 4780 Socialville-Fosters Road, Mason, OH 45040, USA
* Corresponding author. Department of Pulmonary Medicine, University Hospital Antwerp, Wilrijkstraat 10 B-2650, Edegem, Belgium.
E-mail address: wilfried.de.backer@uza.be (W. De Backer).

1556-407X/07/$ – see front matter © 2007 Elsevier Inc. All rights reserved.
sleep.theclinics.com

doi:10.1016/j.jsmc.2007.08.002

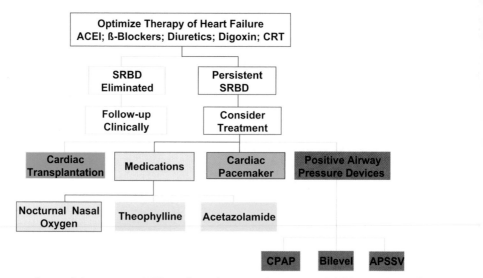

Fig. 1. Treatment of central sleep apnea. ACEI, angiotensin-converting enzyme inhibitor; APSSV, adaptive pressure support servoventilation; CPAP, continuous positive airway pressure; CRT, cardiac resynchronization therapy; SRBD, sleep-related breathing disorder. (*Adapted from* Javaheri S. Sleep-related breathing disorders in heart failure. In: Mann DL, editor. Heart failure: a companion to Braunwald's Heart Disease. Philadelphia: Saunders; 2004. p. 471–87; with permission.)

apnea in the general population and in patients with heart failure [13–15]. These devices are the treatment of choice. Overnight application of nasal CPAP results in a significant decrease in obstructive sleep apnea and arterial oxyhemoglobin desaturation [13], and long-term treatment (1–3 months) results in an increase in left ventricular ejection fraction by about 5% to 10% in heart failure patients with depressed ejection fraction [14,15]. Another study [16] of small numbers (n = 7) of subjects with systolic heart failure showed that 6 weeks of therapy with CPAP significantly increased left

ventricular ejection fraction from 35% to 43%, and improved myocardial efficiency. These parameters did not change in the control group, which consisted of five heart failure patients without OSA.

In contrast, in a randomized double blind (using a placebo CPAP) crossover study [17], no significant changes were observed in left ventricular ejection fraction after 6 weeks of CPAP use. Although, the design of this study [17] was superior to previous studies [14,15] in having a true placebo (sham CPAP), the average nightly use of CPAP was only 3 hours, which was much less than the 5 and 6 hours in the other studies [14,15]. It is therefore likely, that adherence with CPAP is of utmost importance for improvement in cardiac function. This observation is similar to that in patients with hypertension, which only improves with adequate control of sleep apnea [18] and adherence to the use of CPAP [19]. Finally, a recent study [20] showed OSA is associated with significant ($P = .03$) mortality, whereas death did not occur during the follow-up period in heart failure patients who were treated with CPAP with a trend toward significance ($P = .07$), even though "n" was small.

For subjects who do not tolerate high expiratory pressure, bilevel pressure devices should be tried. These devices allow a lower expiratory than inspiratory pressure; therefore, it is easier to exhale. An overnight titration is necessary to determine appropriate level of inspiratory and expiratory pressures.

For subjects with heart failure who cannot tolerate positive pressure devices in spite of consultation with a sleep specialist, nocturnal nasal oxygen or

---

Box 1:   Treatment of obstructive sleep apnea

Aggressive therapy of heart failure, if applicable
Improve sleep hygiene, if applicable
Avoidance of alcoholic beverages, benzodiazepines, narcotics, and sildenafil, particularly at bedtime
Cessation of smoking
Weight reduction, if applicable
Avoidance of supine position in subset of patients with positional OSA (Snore-ball, T-shirt)
Treatment of nasal congestion and obstruction
Nasal positive airway pressure devices
Oral appliances
Nocturnal use of supplemental oxygen
Upper airway surgery
Tracheostomy

For details of treatment of obstructive sleep apnea see the text and Refs. [3,4].

oral appliances may be used. Oral appliances have been effective in treating mild to moderate OSA in the general population. They have also been used to treat sleep apnea in patients with heart failure [21]. From that study [21], however, it was not clear whether the patients had predominately OSA or CSA. The rationale for use of nocturnal supplemental nasal oxygen is to improve periodic breathing and hypoxemia. Improvement in periodic breathing [22] could result in a decrease in obstructive disordered breathing events that occur at the nadir of ventilation [23]. The dose of supplemental nasal oxygen should be determined in the sleep laboratory and varies from 1 to 41 per minute. The dose should be sufficient to eliminate desaturation. Minimizing desaturation and hypoxemia or reoxygenation may have important therapeutic implications.

In summary, there are a number of therapeutic options to treat OSA in heart failure (see Box 1). Positive airway pressure devices are the treatment of choice. All attempts should be exercised to have the patients adhere to these devices, as adherence is critical. Meanwhile, the authors emphasize that no systematic long-term studies are available, and perhaps a randomized study is unethical. However, based on studies of OSA in the general population, the potential consequences of OSA on the cardiovascular system, and limited favorable therapeutic studies using positive airway pressure devices in OSA and heart failure, the authors strongly advise treatment of OSA (even mild cases), with a positive airway device, in heart failure. The hope is to prevent progression of left ventricular remodeling, and perhaps even reverse the remodeling associated with heart failure.

Treatment of central sleep apnea

Treatment of CSA is more difficult than that of obstructive sleep apnea [1,2]. Response to various therapeutic options in general is inhomgeneous (see Fig. 1), with some patients responding well and others not at all. This is true with use of CPAP [13], an observation that is in contrast to the therapeutic effect of CPAP in OSA. A heart failure patient with obstructive sleep apnea can be easily treated with CPAP during an overnight titration process: by the early morning hours, OSA is virtually eliminated [13].

Optimization of cardiopulmonary function

Since central sleep apnea is caused by systolic heart failure; treatment of heart failure either eliminates or improves it. Ultimate treatment of systolic heart failure by cardiac transplantation virtually eliminates central sleep apnea.

The authors suggest intensive therapy of heart failure with diuretics, angiotensin converting enzyme inhibitors (ACEI), and β-blockers before subjecting a patient to sleep study. Improvements in cardiovascular function may even eliminate central sleep apnea [4–8,24]. Beta-blockers are helpful in improving periodic breathing in systolic heart failure. Furthermore, an additional beneficial effect of β-blockers may relate to their counter-balancing of nocturnal cardiac sympathetic hyperactivity caused by sleep apnea. However, β-blockers may adversely affect sleep duration because of their effect on melatonin. Synthesis and secretion of melatonin, a sleep promoting chemical, is via adrenergic signal transduction system. By inhibiting this process, β-blockers, except carvedilol, decrease melatonin secretion [24–26].

Cardiac transplantation

Cardiac transplantation virtually eliminates central sleep apnea. This is not surprising because heart failure is the cause of central sleep apnea. However, with time, a large number of cardiac transplant recipients develop obstructive sleep apnea. This is because of weight gain, which is in part caused by the use of corticosteroids. In the authors' study [27] of 45 cardiac transplant recipients, 36% had an apnea-hypopnea index of more than or equal to 15 per hour. This group of subjects had gained the most weight since transplantation. Obstructive sleep apnea was associated with systemic hypertension and poor quality of life. The authors therefore recommend that cardiac transplant recipients be monitored for development of obstructive sleep apnea. Appropriate dietary regimen to prevent weight gain is prudent, to prevent development of OSA in cardiac transplant recipients. Cardiac transplant patients with obesity should have a sleep study to rule out OSA.

Positive airway pressure devices

Several devices, including CPAP, bilevel, and adaptive pressure support servo-ventilation (APSSV) have been used to treat CSA in patients with systolic heart failure [3,4,28]. However, therapeutic response to these devices is not uniform. In the authors' study [13], first night use of CPAP eliminated central sleep apnea in only 43% of the subjects with systolic heart failure. The remaining subjects (57%) were considered CPAP-nonresponsive. Typically, CPAP-responders needed low level CPAP (6 cm H_2O–10 cm H_2O). In these subjects, the average apnea-hypopnea index decreased from 36 to 4 per hour. In these patients (and in contrast to CPAP nonresponders), the number of premature ventricular contractions, couplets, and ventricular tachycardia decreased (the last was not statistically significant), suggesting a cause and effect relationship. This effect was presumed to be caused by decreased sympathetic activity as arousals decreased and saturation improved.

Heart failure patients with severe central sleep apnea (57% of the subjects) did not respond to acute CPAP titration, and in these subjects ventricular arrhythmias persisted [13]. Several other negative studies have been reported [29–32].

In contrast, several early trials performed in Toronto consistently showed reduction in apnea-hypopnea index, improved desaturation, decreased plasma and urinary norepinephrine, and an increase in left ventricular ejection fraction and mortality [33,34]. Unfortunately, a long-term multicenter Canadian study failed to show any significant effect on mortality [35]. Briefly, in this trial, 258 subjects with heart failure were randomized to CPAP (n = 128) and a control group (n = 130). The average age of 63 years, the left ventricular ejection fraction of 25% and apnea-hypopnea index of 40 per hour, and a minimum saturation of 81% were typical features of heart failure patients with central sleep apnea. The use of CPAP resulted in approximately a 50% reduction the apnea-hypopnea index, considerable improvement in desaturation, and increase in left ventricular ejection fraction. Unfortunately, however, after the first 200 subjects had been followed for a minimum of 6 months and an average follow-up of 2 years, the trial was terminated by the Safety Monitoring Committee. There was increased early mortality with the use of CPAP when compared with the control group (P = .02). After about 3 years, survival favored the CPAP group, but the difference was not as significant (P = .06). The authors have discussed the reasons for CPAP-induced increased mortality, which are multiple [36] and primarily relate to potential adverse hemo-dynamic effects of increased intrathoracic pressure, particularly in patients who are not CPAP responders [13]. In this regard, in a later post-hoc analysis, it was indeed observed that it was CPAP nonresponsiveness that resulted in excess mortality. Survival of CPAP responders improved significantly [37].

Another positive airway pressure device is APSSV. This system acts like a buffer to maintain relatively stable breathing (buffer PAP). This device provides varying amounts of ventilatory support during different phases of periodic breathing. The support is proportional, and is minimal during the hyperpneic phase of periodic breathing and maximal during periods of diminished breathing. In addition, the device will deliver a breath if needed, which prevents development of a central apnea. This variable and proportional support should make this device easier to use and superior to CPAP, because the latter device provides constant positive airway pressure throughout the cycle of periodic breathing. Buffer PAP devices should be optimal to treat sleep related breathing disorders in patients with heart failure, as such patients commonly have a mixture of both obstructive and central apnea. With this device, the expiratory pressure is set at a level to eliminate obstructive apneas and appropriate amount of support is delivered to treat hypopneas. Further, the device is programmed to deliver a breath when needed.

There are now several studies using APSSV systems to treat central sleep apnea in congestive heart failure, all with favorable results [38–42]. APSSV devices may be particularly helpful in those heart failure patients with severe central sleep apnea who may be noncompliant with or nonresponsive to CPAP devices. In this context, the authors have observed [13] that in about 60% of patients with heart failure, CPAP was not therapeutically effective and central sleep apnea persisted. The authors optimistically hypothesize that systematic long-term studies with buffer PAP devices will prove effective in treatment of CSA and result in improved survival of patients with heart failure.

Cardiac pacemakers

A set of different cardiac pacemakers have been used to treat sleep apnea. The authors conclude that pacemakers are generally ineffective for OSA, but to some extent may improve CSA [43–45].

In a study [41] of 15 subjects who had permanent atrial-synchronized ventricular pacemakers placed for symptomatic sinus bradycardia, atrial overdrive (average 72 beats per minute versus spontaneous 57 beats per minute) moderately but significantly decreased the apnea-hypopnea index (from 28 to 11 per hour), improved arterial oxyhemoglobin desaturation, and decreased arousals. These patients had predominantly mild to moderate central sleep apnea, and some of them had mild left ventricular systolic dysfunction. Two other studies [42,43] suggest that ventricular pacing improved CSA in a subset of subjects. The mechanisms for improvement of sleep apnea with pacemakers are perhaps related to increased cardiac output and decreased pulmonary capillary pressure and right heart pressure (increasing upper airway size). If these assumptions are true, in patients with significantly reduced left ventricular ejection fraction, biventricular pacing [46] may be therapeutically more effective in treating CSA than atrial pacing overdrive (in patients with bradycardia). As noted above, pacemakers are ineffective for treatment of OSA.

Medications

A number of medications including oxygen, acetozolamide, and theophylline, have been used to treat

CSA. Supplemental nasal oxygen has been studied the most [47–52].

Nocturnal supplemental nasal oxygen

Systematic studies in patients with systolic heart failure [3,4,22,47–52] have shown that nocturnal therapy with supplemental nasal oxygen improves central sleep apnea. The dose of oxygen should be determined by an overnight study and should be sufficient to eliminate desaturation. One study has shown that treatment of CSA with oxygen decreases muscle sympathetic nerve activity [51], and two randomized, placebo controlled, double-blind studies have shown that short-term (1–4 weeks) administration of nocturnal supplemental nasal oxygen improves maximum exercise capacity [50] and decreases overnight urinary norepinephrine excretion [49]. Furthermore, in a recent randomized (open) study, Sasayama and colleagues [52] reported that nocturnal administration of nasal oxygen for 9 weeks improved sleep apnea, desaturation, and resulted in significant improvement in left ventricular ejection fraction and quality of life of heart failure patients. These improvements were not observed in the control group. The improvement in left ventricular ejection fraction is of critical importance because it is a predictor of survival of heart failure patients. In another study [53], administration of oxygen resulted in improvement of sleep apnea, desaturation, and brain naturetic peptide.

In spite of the above studies, prospective, placebo controlled long-term studies are necessary [22] to determine if nocturnal oxygen therapy has the potential to decrease morbidity and mortality of patients with systolic heart failure.

Theophylline

It has long been known that theophylline is a respiratory stimulant and is helpful to treat central apnea both in infants and in adults. Open studies [54,55] and a randomized, double blind, placebo-controlled study [56] have shown the efficacy of theophylline in the treatment of central sleep apnea in heart failure. In this crossover study [56] of 15 subjects with treated, stable systolic heart failure, oral theophylline at therapeutic plasma concentration (11 μg/ml, range 7 μg/ml–15 μg/ml), decreased the apnea-hypopnea index by about 50% and improved arterial oxyhemoglobin saturation. Potential arrhythmogenic effects and phosphodiesterase inhibition are common concerns with long-term use of theophylline in patients with heart failure. However, there are no long-term controlled studies. If theophylline is used to treat CSA, frequent and careful follow-ups are necessary.

Mechanisms of action of theophylline in improving central apnea remain unclear [57]. However, at therapeutic serum concentrations, theophylline competes with adenosine at some of its receptor sites. In the central nervous system, adenosine is a respiratory depressant and theophylline stimulates respiration [57–59] by competing with adenosine. Conceivably, therefore, an increase in ventilation by theophylline could decrease CSA.

Acetazolamide

Acetazolamide is a mild diuretic and a respiratory stimulant and has been used for treatment for prevention and treatment of periodic breathing at high altitude. It has also been used for treatment of idiopathic CSA [60,61]. In a recent double blind, placebo-controlled crossover study [62] of 12 subjects with heart failure, acetazolamide administered at about 3 mg/kg one half hour before bedtime, decreased the central apnea-hypopnea index significantly from about 57 per hour (in the placebo arm) to 34 per hour. Acetazolamide improved arterial oxyhemoglobin desaturation significantly. Furthermore patients reported improved subjective perception of overall sleep quality, feeling rested on awakening, falling asleep unintentionally during daytime, and fatigue. Acetazolamide, therefore, could have other advantageous effects when used in patients with heart failure and central sleep apnea, including acting as a mild diuretic and also normalizing the alkalemia (caused by loop diuretics) commonly present in patients with heart failure. In the authors' patients, arterial blood pH decreased from 7.43 to 7.37.

Summary

There are no guidelines for the treatment of sleep apnea in heart failure. CSA remains difficult to treat. Well-designed, long-term controlled studies are needed to determine if any treatment prolongs survival. No such studies are also available for treatment of CSA or OSA in heart failure. However, based on pathophysiologic consequences of sleep apnea on the cardiovascular system, studies associating excess mortality of heart failure patients with CSA and OSA, and limited favorable therapeutic studies, the authors suggest identifying heart failure patients who may suffer from sleep apnea and treating them appropriately.

References

[1] Javaheri S, Parker TJ, Wexler L, et al. Occult sleep-disordered breathing in stable congestive heart failure. Ann Intern Med 1995;122:487–92. Published erratum appears in Ann Intern Med 1995;123:77.

[2] Javaheri S, Parker TJ, Liming JD, et al. Sleep apnea in 81 ambulatory male patients with stable

heart failure: types and their prevalence's, consequences, and presentations. Circulation 1998;97: 2154–9. This is the largest prospective and most systematic study of patients with systolic heart failure.

[3] Javaheri S. Sleep disorders in systolic heart failure: a prospective study of 100 male patients. The final report. Int J Cardiol 2006;106:21–8.

[4] Javaheri S. Heart failure. In: Kryger MH, Roth T, Dement WC, editors. Principles and practice of sleep medicine. 4th edition. Philadelphia: WB Saunders; 2005. This is the most updated article regarding sleep related breathing disorders in heart failure.

[5] Javaheri S. Sleep-related breathing disorders in heart failure. In: Mann DL, editor. Heart failure, a companion to Braunwald's heart disease. Philadelphia: WB Saunders; 2004. p. 471–87. This article reviews cardiovascular consequences of sleep apnea in heart failure.

[6] Javaheri S, Wexler L. Prevalence and treatment of breathing disorders during sleep in heart failure patients. Curr Treat Options Cardiovasc Med 2005;7:295–305.

[7] Wexler L, Javaheri S. Sleep apnea in heart failure: epidemiology and treatment. Cleve Clin J Med 2005;72:929–36.

[8] Javaheri S. Central sleep apnea in congestive heart failure: prevalence, mechanisms, impact and therapeutic options. Seminars in Respiratory and Critical Care Medicine 2005;25:44–55.

[9] Shepard JW Jr, Pevernagie DA, Stanson AW, et al. Effects of changes in central venous pressure on upper airway size in patients with obstructive sleep apnea. Am J Respir Crit Care Med 1996; 153:250–4.

[10] Calle EE, Thun MJ, Petrelli JM, et al. Body-mass index and mortality in a prospective cohort of U.S. adults. N Engl J Med 1999;341:1097–105.

[11] Kenchaiah S, Evans JC, Levy D, et al. Obesity and the risk of heart failure. N Engl J Med 2002;347: 305–13.

[12] Roizenblatt S, Guilleminault C, Poyares D, et al. A double-blind study of sildenafil in obstructive sleep apnea. Arch Intern Med 2006; 166:1763–7.

[13] Javaheri S. Effects of continuous positive airway pressure on sleep apnea and ventricular irritability in patients with heart failure. Circulation 2000;101:392–7.

[14] Mansfield DR, Gollogly C, Kaye DM. Controlled trail of continuous positive airway pressure in obstructive sleep apnea and heart failure. Am J Respir Crit Care Med 2004;169:361–6.

[15] Kaneko Y, Floras JS, Usui K, et al. Cardiovascular effects of continuous positive airway pressure in patients with heart failure and obstructive sleep apnea. N Engl J Med 2003;248:1233–41.

[16] Yoshinaga K, Burwash I, Leech J, et al. The effects of continuous positive airway pressure on myocardial energetics in patients with heart failure

and obstructive sleep apnea. J Am Coll Cardiol 2007;49:450–8.

[17] Smith L, Vennelle M, Garder R, et al. Auto-titrating continuous positive airway pressure therapy in patients with chronic heart failure and obstructive sleep apnea: a randomized placebo-controlled trial. Eur Heart J 2007;28:1221–7.

[18] Becker H, Jerrentrup A, Ploch T, et al. Effect of nasal continuous positive airway pressure treatment on blood pressure in patients with obstructive sleep apnea. Circulation 2003;107:68–73.

[19] Faccenda J, Mackay T, Boon N, et al. Randomized placebo-controlled trial of continuous positive airway pressure on blood pressure in the sleep apnea-hypopnea syndrome. Am J Respir Crit Care Med 2001;163:344–8.

[20] Wang H, Parker J, Newton G, et al. Influence of obstructive sleep apnea on mortality in patients with heart failure. J Am Coll Cardiol 2007; 49(15):1625–31.

[21] Eskafi M. Sleep apnea in patients with stable congestive heart failure. Swed Dent J Suppl 2004; 168:1–107.

[22] Javaheri S. Pembrey's Dream: the time has come for a long-term trial of nocturnal supplemental nasal oxygen to treat central sleep apnea in congestive heart failure. Chest 2003;123:322–5.

[23] Hudgel D, Chapman KR, Franks C, et al. Changes in inspiratory muscle electrical activity and upper airway resistance during periodic breathing induced by hypoxemia during sleep. Am Rev Respir Dis 1987;135:899–906.

[24] Solin P, Bergin P, Richardson M, et al. Influence of pulmonary capillary wedge pressure on central apnea in heart failure. Circulation 1999;99: 1574–9.

[25] Arendt J, Bojkowski C, Franey C, et al. Immunoassay of 6-hydroxymelatonin sulfate in human plasma and urine: abolition of the urinary 24-hour rhythm with atenolol. J Clin Endocrinol Metab 1985;60:1166–73.

[26] Stoschitzky K, Sakotnik A, Lercher P, et al. Influence of beta-blockers on melatonin release. Eur J Clin Pharmacol 1999;55:111–5.

[27] Javaheri S, Abraham W, Brown C, et al. Prevalence of obstructive sleep apnea and periodic limb movements in 45 subjects with heart transplantation. Eur Heart J 2004;25:260–6.

[28] Javaheri S. Heart failure and sleep apnea: emphasis on practical therapeutic options. Clin Chest Med 2003;24:207–22. This is a review article regarding use of positive pressure airway devices in patients with heart failure and various types of sleep apnea.

[29] Guilleminault C, Clerk A, Labanowski M, et al. Cardiac failure and benzodiazepines. Sleep 1993;16:524–8.

[30] Davies RJO, Harrington KJ, Ormerod JM, et al. Nasal continuous positive airway pressure in chronic heart failure with sleep-disordered breathing. Am Rev Respir Dis 1993;147:630–4.

[31] Buckle P, Millar T, Kryger M. The effects of short-term nasal CPAP on Cheyne-Stokes respiration in congestive heart failure. Chest 1992;102:31–5.

[32] Keily JL, Deegan P, Buckley A, et al. Efficacy of nasal continuous positive airway pressure therapy in chronic heart failure: importance of underlying cardiac rhythm. Thorax 1998;53:956–62.

[33] Sin DD, Logan AG, Fitzgerald FS, et al. Effects of continuous positive airway pressure on cardiovascular outcomes in heart failure patients with and without Cheyne-Stokes respiration. Circulation 2000;102:61–6.

[34] Naughton MT, Bernard DC, Liu PP, et al. Effects of nasal CPAP on sympathetic activity in patients with heart failure and central sleep apnea. Am J Respir Crit Care Med 1995;152:473–9.

[35] Bradley T, Logan A, Kimoff J, et al. Continuous positive airway pressure for central sleep apnea and heart failure. N Engl J Med 2006;353:2025–33.

[36] Javaheri S. CPAP should not be used for central sleep apnea in congestive heart failure patients. J Clin Sleep Med 2006;2(4):399–402.

[37] Arzt M, Floras JS, Logan AG, et al. Suppression of central sleep apnea by continuous positive air pressure and transplant-free survival in heart failure. Circulation 2007;115:3173–80.

[38] Teschler H, Döhring J, Wang YM. Adaptive pressure support servo-ventilation: a novel treatment for Cheyne-Stokes respiration in heart failure. Am J Respir Crit Care Med 2001;64:614–9.

[39] Pepperell J, Maskell N, Jones D, et al. A randomized controlled trial of adaptive ventilation for Cheyne-Stokes breathing in heart failure. Am J Respir Crit Care Med 2003;168:1109–14.

[40] Szollosi I, O'driscoll D, Dayer M, et al. Adaptive servo-ventilation and dead space: effects on central sleep apnoea. J Sleep Res 2006;15:199–205.

[41] Philippe C, Stoica-Herman M, Drouot X, et al. Compliance with and effectiveness of adaptive servoventilation versus continuous positive airway pressure in the treatment of Cheyne-Stokes respiration in heart failure over a six month period. Heart 2006;92:337–42.

[42] Kasai T, Narui K, Dohi T, et al. First experience of using new adaptive servo-ventilation device for Cheyne-Stokes respiration with central sleep apnea among Japanese patients with congestive heart failure. Circ J 2006;70:1148–54.

[43] Garrigue S, Bordier P, Jaïs P, et al. Benefit of atrial pacing in sleep apnea syndrome. N Engl J Med 2002;346:404–12.

[44] Sinha A, Skobel E, Breithardt O, et al. Cardiac resynchronization therapy improves central sleep apnea and Cheyne-Stokes respiration in patients with chronic heart failure. J Am Coll Cardiol 2004;44:68–71.

[45] Gabor J, Newman D, Barnard-Roberts V, et al. Improvement in Cheyne-Stokes respiration following cardiac resynchronization therapy. Eur Respir J 2006;26:95–100.

[46] Abraham WT, Hayes DL. Cardiac resynchronization therapy for heart failure. Circulation 2004;108:2596–603.

[47] Hanly PF, Millar TW, Steljes DG, et al. The effect of oxygen on respiration and sleep in patients with congestive heart failure. Ann Intern Med 1989;111:777–82.

[48] Javaheri S, Ahmed M, Parker TJ, et al. Effects of nasal O2 on sleep-related disordered breathing in ambulatory patients with stable heart failure. Sleep 1999;22:1101–6.

[49] Staniforth AD, Kinneart WJM, Hetmanski DJ, et al. Effect of oxygen on sleep quality, cognitive function and sympathetic activity in patients with chronic heart failure and Cheyne-Stokes respiration. Eur Heart J 1998;19:922–8.

[50] Andreas S, Clemens C, Sandholzer H, et al. Improvement of exercise capacity with treatment of Cheyne-Stokes respiration in patients with congestive heart failure. J Am Coll Cardiol 1996;27:1486–90.

[51] Andreas S, Bingeli C, Mohacsi P, et al. Nasal oxygen and muscle sympathetic nerve activity in heart failure. Chest 2003;123:366–71. This study confirms the results of Ref. [31] using peroneal nerve sympathetic activity.

[52] Sasayama S, Izumi T, Seino Y, et al. Effects of nocturnal oxygen therapy on outcome measures in patients with chronic heart failure and Cheyne-Stokes respiration. Circ J 2006;70:1–7.

[53] Shigemitsu M, Nishio K, Kusuyama T, et al. Nocturnal oxygen therapy prevents progress of congestive heart failure with central sleep apnea. Int J Cardiol 2007;115:354–60.

[54] Dowdell WT, Javaheri S, McGinnis W. Cheyne-Stokes respiration presenting as sleep apnea syndrome. Clinical and polysomnographic features. Am Rev Respir Dis 1990;141:871–9.

[55] Ke H, Qingquan L, Jiong Y, et al. The effect of theophylline on sleep-disordered breathing in patients with stable chronic congestive heart failure. Chin Med J 2003;116:1711–6.

[56] Javaheri S, Parker TJ, Wexler L, et al. Effect of theophylline on sleep-disordered breathing in heart failure. N Engl J Med 1996;335:562–7.

[57] Javaheri S, Teppama LJ, Evers JAM. Effects of aminophylline on hypoxemia-induced ventilatory depression in cats. J Appl Physiol 1988;64:1837–43.

[58] Javaheri S, Evers JAM, Teppema LJ. Increase in ventilation caused by aminophylline in the absence of changes in ventral extracellular fluid pH and PCO2. Thorax 1989;44:121–5.

[59] Javaheri S, Guerra LF. Lung function, hypoxic and hypercapnic ventilatory responses, and respiratory muscle strength in normal subjects taking oral theophylline. Thorax 1990;45:743–7.

[60] DeBacker W, Berbraecken J, Willemen M, et al. Central apnea index decreases after prolonged treatment with acetazolamide. Am J Respir Crit Care Med 1995;151:87–91.

[61] Verbraecken J, Willemen M, DeCock W, et al. Central sleep apnea after interrupting long-term acetazolamide therapy. Respir Physiol 1998;112: 57–70.

[62] Javaheri S. Acetazolamide Improves Central Sleep Apnea in heart failure. A double-blind prospective study. Am J Respir Crit Care Med 2006; 173:234–7.

SLEEP
MEDICINE
CLINICS

Sleep Med Clin 2 (2007) 639–642

Index

Note: Page numbers of article titles are in **boldface** type.

A

Acetazolamide, for treatment of central sleep apnea in heart failure patients, 635

Apnea. *See* Central sleep apnea (CSA) *and* Obstructive sleep apnea (OSA).

Apneic threshold, and ventilatory response to CO_2 below eupnea during sleep, 634–635

Arrhythmia, OSA and, **575–581**
> atrial fibrillation, 577
> bradyarrhythmias, 576–577
> mechanisms of, 575–576
> sudden cardiac death, 578
> treatment, 578–579
> ventricular ectopy and arrhythmias, 577–578
> risk factor or association with stroke, 587

Atherosclerosis, in OSA, risk factor or association with stroke, 587–588

Atrial fibrillation, OSA and, 577

B

Blood coagulation abnormalities, leading to cardiovascular disease in OSA, 542–543

Blood pressure, effects of OSA on, 550–551
> daytime, 550–551
> nighttime, 550
> physiologic effects of sleep on, 550

Bradyarrhythmias, OSA and, 576–577

Breathing, control of, 623–624
> periodic, mechanisms of, in systolic heart failure, **623–630**

Burnout, cardiovascular implications of, 534–535

C

Cardiac arrhythmia, in OSA, risk factor or association with stroke, 587

Cardiac pacemakers, for treatment of CSA in heart failure patients, 634

Cardiac transplantation, for treatment of CSA in heart failure patients, 633

Cardiopulmonary function, optimization of, for treatment of CSA in heart failure patients, 633

Cardiovascular disease, implications of poor sleep, **529–538**
> burnout or vital exhaustion, 534–535
> cardiovascular measures, 529–530
> heart disease, 531–532
> hypertension, 530–531
> sleep deprivation and restriction, 532–534
> sleep fragmentation, 535

in OSA, arrhythmias, **575–581**
> coronary artery disease and, **559–564**
> heart failure, **631–638**
> left ventricular systolic and diastolic dysfunction, **565–574**
> mortality in, **593–601**
> pathophysiologic mechanisms of, **539–547**
>> blood coagulation abnormalities, 542–543
>> endothelial dysfunction, 541
>> glucose intolerance, 543
>> inflammation, 541–542
>> leptin pathway, 543
>> metabolic dysregulation, 543
>> oxidative stress, 541
>> sympathetic nervous system overactivity, 540–541
> stroke and, **583–591**
> systemic and pulmonary arterial hypertension in, **549–557**

1556-407X/07/$ – see front matter © 2007 Elsevier Inc. All rights reserved.
sleep.theclinics.com

doi:10.1016/S1556-407X(07)00131-2

Moving?

Make sure your subscription moves with you!

To notify us of your new address, find your **Clinics Account Number** (located on your mailing label above your name), and contact customer service at:

E-mail: elspcs@elsevier.com

800-654-2452 (subscribers in the U.S. & Canada)
407-345-4000 (subscribers outside of the U.S. & Canada)

Fax number: 407-363-9661

Elsevier Periodicals Customer Service
6277 Sea Harbor Drive
Orlando, FL 32887-4800

*To ensure uninterrupted delivery of your subscription, please notify us at least 4 weeks in advance of move.

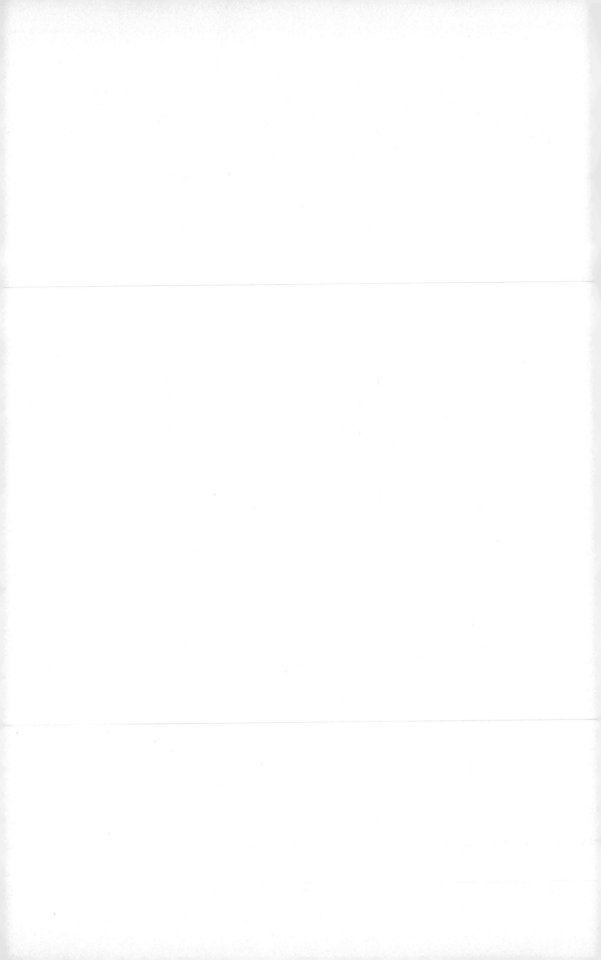